Rare *but* not Alone

Raising Kids *with* Cyclic Vomiting Syndrome

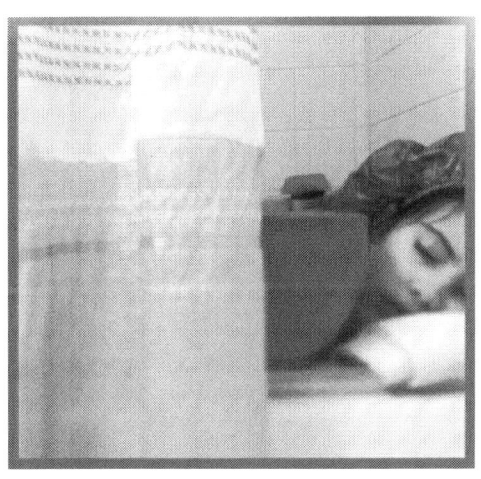

COLLEEN RICE

Copyright © 2014 by Colleen Rice
Cover photo by Dar Sanchez

All rights reserved. No part of this publication may be reproduced, distributed, or transmitted in any form or by any means, including photocopying, recording, or other electronic or mechanical methods, without the prior written permission of the author, except in the case of brief quotations embodied in critical reviews and certain other noncommercial uses permitted by copyright law. For permission requests, write to the author, addressed "Attention: Permissions" at the email address below.

RareButNotAlone@gmail.com
www.rarebutnotalone.com

Opinions expressed by contributors are their own and not necessarily those of Rare But Not Alone (RBNA) author Colleen Rice or Cyclic Vomiting Association (CVSA). RBNA and CVSA do not endorse any specific product, medication, treatment or claim by a contributor and disclaims all liability relating thereto. The content of the Rare But Not Alone Raising Kids with Cyclic Vomiting Syndrome is for education purposes and in no way intended to replace the knowledge of your doctor. We advise working closely with a physician in regard to a patient's health care needs.

Acknowledgements

Dedicated to my family: My parents Donald and Peg Badger, my husband Daniel, and our children, Matthew, Kate, Andrew, Greg, Lauren and Julianne. CVS is a family affair and impacts everyone. Thank you for your patience.....

Special thanks to the Cyclic Vomiting Syndrome Association, USA, without which we would still be fumbling in the dark.....

Special thanks to all my CVS mom and dad friends, who encouraged me along the way to make sure I did not give up on this book.

Contents

Rare But Not Alone.... A Leap of Faith...	9
The CVS Journey	11
The Many Paths to a Diagnosis	43
Finding the Right Treatment Plan For Your Child	85
Riding Out the Storm of a CVS Cycle	105
Making the Plan: Documenting Your Path	132
Choosing a Peaceful Path	137
Family Life	154
The Education Question for CVS kids	181
Raising Awareness and Giving Back	196
The Sky's the Limit for CVS Kids	209
Appendix	215
Cyclic Vomiting Syndrome Association (CVSA) December 2014	215
Extreme Emesis: Cyclic Vomiting Syndrome	218

Foreword

"I opened your book draft and was quite amazed, impressed and grateful to see the extent of your writing, research, persistence and dedication to this project. This is the gift of depth—the ripples are visible only for a short time and then you'll lose sight of the effect you have as they travel outward. You will be reaching those that are still suffering in isolation from Cyclic Vomiting Syndrome. In spite of 22 years of work we are still trying to pull this condition out of the cracks in the floorboard of medicine. Thank you, Colleen."

Kathleen Adams, Founder, President and Research Liaison of CVSA

Breaking the Silence
By Tiffany Sharpe

When I became a mother I didn't think about what could go wrong.
All I could think about was holding her for so long.
Then it started when she was about a year old.
We saw doctor after doctor and no answers were told.
We finally found the right avenue.
Someone who knows what we are going through.

She has to deal with the "pukies" a lot.
She doesn't know any different and doesn't give it a thought.
To her this is normal and that's okay.
We are teaching her to lean on God and her faith.
So when you feel like there's nowhere to turn and feel all alone,
Just remember it takes a special person to be the parent of a child with Cyclic Vomiting Syndrome.

Rare But Not Alone.... A Leap of Faith...

■ ■ ■

Why would I write a book on Cyclic Vomiting Syndrome? I am not an author by profession, nor am I in the medical field as a nurse or a doctor. However, I am a parent, entrusted with the caring and raising of a child who has a rare and often misunderstood condition. What you see before you is a labor of love, written in hopes of helping other parents who find themselves in a similar position.

As parents of a child with a rare condition, we are forced to come to terms with the fact that what works for the vast majority of kids who are treated in the ER for throwing up will often not work for us. We take our children to doctors assuming that they know what is making our children sick, and often we find that there are no answers. We travel to see specialists in the fields of gastroenterology, neurology, and genetics, and few know how to help us. If we are blessed we might find one who has personal experience with CVS, either knowing someone who has it or having had it themselves.

It is my hope that this book will become a way to define us as community, and say to the world that CVS is not in our children's heads and they are not making themselves sick. The cornerstone of our community is the Cyclic Vomiting Association, which was founded as a leap of faith by a mother in search of answers for her child. I'm sure Kathleen Adams, back in 1990s, was taking a huge step out into the unknown at the time and was also unable to fathom what her decision to embrace this cause would mean to the world. Could she have failed and given up? Yes, but she stuck with it, overcoming numerous challenges set before her. Her searching has helped thousands of other parents on the same journey. It was her labor of love for our community. I will be forever grateful for all the sacrifices she has made.

Awareness of CVS is growing each day as more and more children are being correctly diagnosed. It is often the frustrated and desperate parents who discover the diagnosis by searching the internet for answers. This often comes after years of numerous emergency room visits and the brush off of the vomiting being "just another virus." Parents of children with CVS know there is more to this evil sickness, and it is robbing our kids of a joyful childhood and until now no one has written our stories to share with the world what our life is like.

Any journey is better when you do not have to go it alone. Imagine that you are lost in a foreign country, not knowing the language, or how to get to where you want to go. This is what parents of a children with CVS felt only a generation ago, and many still feel this way today. Today parents are blessed to have a roadmap to help navigate the twists and turns and obstacles as they arise. Today there is a wealth of resources available and a wide variety of treatment options.

Within this book you will find the experiences of parents just like yourself trying to make the best life possible for their child while living with CVS. It is my hope that you find this book to be a general roadmap, and also a source of comfort and validation as well as a resource to share with those around you. The CVS families whose stories are in this book come from eight different countries and with children ranging from infants on up to college age and beyond. They shared my desire to raise awareness in speaking out so that others will no longer feel so alone. On March 5, 2015 we will celebrate our first worldwide CVS awareness day and raise even more awareness than in the past. When we share our stories, we tell the world that though we are rare, we are not alone.

Colleen Rice

The CVS Journey

In Search of a Caregiver

While I was speaking with a fellow CVS mom, Danica Martin, we thought it would be fun to make a list of the job skills that a CVS parent would have. Neither of us were really prepared for life as a CVS parent during the early days. I only had a slight advantage, having lived with undiagnosed CVS in my own childhood. We swapped horror stories and honor stories. We shared accounts about the awful cycles our kids had been through. We validated each other's challenges in ways only a parent who has been there could. We both wished there was a handbook that came along with the rare diagnosis. Neither of us had anyone we could to turn to for advice on how to raise a child with this unique health disorder. Together we came up with hypothetical job description for a CVS parent, including many tasks a CVS parent takes on:

Job requirements for a CVS Parent.

1. Be willing to be your child's greatest advocate. Be ready to fight for your child's needs in order to keep them well.
2. Be willing to sleep with "one eye open" in case a cycle hits at night. Some children have a hard time calling for a parent when the vomiting starts in the early hours of the morning. Key onset times are typically between 3-6 am. Must be prepared to respond at any given moment to the sound of forceful vomiting.
3. You may need to think creatively about how to catch vomit, such as in a bucket, towel, or any other acceptable means to avoid

massive clean-up. This may mean storing things in various places for quick access. For example, a puke bucket or towel under each bed or in every bathroom. Some parents choose special buckets or cups for their child to always have as their own personal puke catcher. Must be willing to do LOTS and LOTS of laundry.

4. Be prepared to keep diaries detailing each episode, including start and end time, treating doctors and nurses, foods consumed, and timing and quantity of input and output. If your child's episodes are mild or infrequent this might seem unnecessary; however, tracking allows you and your doctors to understand the bigger picture of your child's episodes, triggers and intensity. Our advice: track the exact date of child's episode, length of episode, and the interval between episodes. Also record the name and effectiveness of each medication administered in order to present a clear picture of what does and does not work well for your child.

5. Be ready to know the names of all sorts of medications and supplements. In the next few years you will feel like a pharmacist, particularly when it comes to anti-nausea medicines. Helpful hint: teaching your child the names of the medications can be very helpful as well so that they can ask for the specific ones depending on how they are feeling and help empower them when they are older and responsible caring for themselves.

6. Be prepared to learn the idiosyncrasies of the CVS world. You will come to know key terms such as "preventative" and "abort," the latter term meaning to stop a cycle once it has started or is in full swing.

7. Be willing to be accessible by phone at all times. An older CVS child will appreciate knowing that your phone is always nearby in case an episode begins while he or she is at school, on a play date, or with a babysitter. A CVS parent is also often waiting for return phone calls from doctors.

8. A CVS parent should have a treatment plan in case an episode begins while you are not with your child. Be ready to explain

CVS to unfamiliar nurses, teachers, relatives and others who are involved in your child's life. Unfortunately, not everyone will listen to your plan in such a way that makes you feel heard. We have experienced a few CVS non-believers and it is always quite frustrating. Our helpful hint: keep your cool. Vent to other CVS parents if it helps and then continue working hard to make your child's needs known.

9. Be willing to learn the signs of dehydration and realize that it can happen in the span of an hour.
10. Be ready to travel! Unfortunately, there are not many doctors who have been educated regarding Cyclic Vomiting Syndrome. CVS families often make road trips to see a doctor who specializes in cyclic vomiting syndrome. Our helpful hint: make an appointment with the best doctor you can find and plan a vacation around appointments! Save for trips to Wisconsin or other "exotic" places instead of Disney World.
11. Be willing to work closely with insurance companies. Remind case managers that you are doing your best to improve the health of your child. They don't want to spend unnecessary money on your sick child and you don't want your child to be sick. You are working together!

You may have found yourself thrown into this job even without the above mentioned skills. Don't forget: the only absolute qualification is love for your child and a willingness to learn.

My CVS Journey: Rare and Alone

It seems like only yesterday I was the one struggling with intense vomiting during the mid 1980s. Everyone knew that when I threw up, I never stopped, but we had no understanding of why. I dry heaved for hours to the point of bile and would lie in what is now called a conscious coma. The doctors never knew what to think when my parent sought help for me. My parents had a pharmacist friend recommended

Emetrol, which only seemed to aggravate the vomiting. If I was finally to be admitted to the hospital (this occurred only three times in my childhood), the nurses told my parents that I was just being stubborn and needed to stop. Emetrol, which only seemed to aggravate the vomiting. If I was finally to be admitted to the hospital (this occurred only three times in my childhood), the nurses told my parents that I was just being stubborn and needed to stop.

We continued to ride out cycles at home rather than be told it was all in my head. Thankfully in my case it only happened 3-4 times a year. I felt guilty. Why could I not throw up like everyone else? Why would the sound of someone flushing the toilet trigger such horrible retching over and over again? Why could I not swallow or take sips and keep them down like everyone else? The problem must be me. I must be weak. Never did it occur to me that this was not normal, that it could be something more. I remember sitting in the doctor's office with my son a week after his diagnosis saying, "Well of course he's sensitive to light and sound, that's normal right?" My son's pediatrician then explained that it was not. I was so shocked to learn, at age 35, that the way I had always experienced throwing up was not the norm. I had long since noticed that Andrew's vomiting would always start around 4:00 am and then kick into high gear once the sun rose, and now I knew why.

My parents did the best they could with the knowledge they had and the resources available to them. The next time we were able get treatment for an episode was in 1991, during which my kidneys were on the verge of shutting down during a seven day episode. My mother refused to be dismissed by the emergency room doctor. Thankfully another doctor who knew my mother well happened to be at the right place at the right time and was able to intervene for me. No one believed her when she told them I had not peed in several days. She knew because she never left my side during the episode. My mom fought for what I needed, as alone as she felt at the time. She did not know what was happening to me or that it had a name, which made it all the scarier.

We were completely unaware at the time that hopeful things were in the works. There was another little girl about my age suffering from

CVS much worse than I. Her mother, Kathleen Adams, had a medical field background and was searching desperately for answers. She was able to get the diagnosis of Cyclic Vomiting Syndrome. In 1993, she urged medical professionals to become more committed to developing a better understanding of CVS. Her hope, which was initially just to help her daughter, grew into an International Support Group that has helped thousands of people young and old. Officials from the Cyclic Vomiting Syndrome Association (CVSA) gathered researchers for the first International Scientific Symposium in 1994. Those present were pediatric gastroenterologists, Dr. David Fleisher and Dr. B U.K. Li, who recognized that clarifications were needed to assist medical professionals in diagnosing CVS.

It would take another 14 years to finalize a consensus statement to help improve the diagnosis and treatment of Cyclic Vomiting Syndrome. In 2007 Dr. Li and Dr. V published in *Practical Gastro* a groundbreaking article "Extreme Emesis" (which can be found in the back of this book). Dr. David Fleisher also published his own *Empirical Guidelines for Treatment of Cyclic Vomiting Syndrome* in April 2008, which still stands as a important resource. In 2008, the North American Society for Pediatric Gastroenterology, Herpetology and Nutrition (NASPGHAN) published the first consensus guidelines for physicians to follow if they suspected a child had CVS. Before this time, it was difficult for a physician to say without a reasonable doubt that a patient had CVS. Included in this statement were diagnostic guidelines and treatment suggestions that would change the world's approach to CVS.

CVS was finally more fully acknowledged as a real medical condition, which offered hope to those suffering. From then on children would have more of chance with these new criteria and awareness. The medical community is still trying to find and understand what causes CVS, and how best to treat it. Theories range from it being a migraine variant to a functional mitochondrial dysfunction. Treatments are typically targeted at managing known triggers or conditions that set off the CVS cycle and having a plan in place to stop cycles once they have started.

Andrew's Path: Repeating History

While my CVS days were in the past, I had to walk that path again, this time as a parent. I remember the whirlwind of the thoughts that I had when we found out we were expecting our third child in the summer of 2006. At the time my husband and I had been married for five years, and already had two children. We were very excited, but wondered if we were ready to be outnumbered. Would our daughter have a sister? Would our son have a brother? Would he or she take after Dad and have blue eyes like our other two children or would I finally get a child with brown eyes like mine? As luck would have it, he inherited my brown eyes along with something else I had never considered. One thought I never had was, what were the chances of him throwing up like I did as a child? I had long since forgotten the vomiting, and had written it off as a personal weakness or character flaw that I had overcome. I had never heard of anyone else suffering the same thing. Never did I imagine that I would one day watch my son go through what I did. However, what was different in his case was that he would get a formal diagnosis of Cyclic Vomiting Syndrome. We would have team of wonderful, knowledgeable doctors and an amazing network of fellow parents to help us through this.

Despite my history of Cyclic Vomiting Syndrome, I never developed Hyperemesis Gravidarum or an intense form of morning sickness, in any of my 6 pregnancies. Oddly enough during pregnancy was the first time in my life that I learned throwing up did not have to be crippling. Three weeks prior to my due date, I went into labor and we welcomed Andrew into our family. I laugh now when I reflect on how Andrew came into the world being pushed out along with intense vomiting, which is common during labor and delivery. Interestingly, he is the only one of my kids during whose delivery I had vomited. He also was our only child to need the Neonatal Intensive Care Unit. When he was born, he had a hard time remembering to breathe and had very low muscle tone. I remember seeing him for only a minute before they rushed him down the hall. He was blue and limp with a glazed look in his eyes and barely responsive. Just after his birth, I was lying in an empty room, as my husband had gone with our new son to see if he was going to be all right. Was he going to live? Would he breathe on his own? A dear friend had shared with me how she got through losing twins by thinking "from the womb to God's arms." That image carried me through as the moments dragged on. Fortunately, it was only a short time, two hours or so before I learned that he was doing better and I would be able to go down there and hold him. He spent a total of five days in the NICU before coming home.

Once Andrew was released from the NICU four days later, things returned to almost normal. He had reflux and we tried a variety of medications that really did not do much. The reflux seemed to come and go and then disappeared. He was an infant who startled easily and loved to be held or swaddled. This came in handy later as nurses often swaddle or wrap kids tightly when putting in IVs. He surprised numerous nurses as he would smile and calm down every time they did this. I knew in the back of my mind something was unique about Andrew and the way in which he physically processed things. When he got sick, he didn't rebound as quickly as his siblings, and he seemed more intense when throwing up. Also when he got fevers they were never low grade but always 104-106 for no known reason.

The older he got, the more pronounced his issues became. At age three, he was hospitalized for strep throat because of the vomiting, but we wrote it off as the tonsils. We had his tonsils removed in December 2010 in hopes of solving this problem, along with his horrific snoring. There were several other emergency room trips between this one and his formal diagnosis. Each time, I just took it as the way he threw up and wrote it off as something he inherited from me. It was something we had to live with as I had in my childhood. I had no idea the level to which this would grow over the coming years.

In April of 2012, things changed. We had gone through a lot as a family leading up to this. My only brother was killed in a car crash the day after Thanksgiving in 2010. No one saw it coming that a young hard working husband and father of two would suddenly be gone. This reminded all of us of the fragility of human life and how you could easily lose it all in the blink of an eye. This was my only brother, my partner in crime so to speak, my best childhood friend, one of my lifelines....and he was gone. I remember the desire to cry each time my husband left each day, fearing that he might not return. I know the kids held on to us a little tighter in the weeks and months following this loss. Their cousins who were close in age to them had lost their father. What if they lost theirs? They also had a lot of "what ifs" running through their young heads, and we could only reassure them as much as we could as we were grappling with the same questions and found no reasonable answers. Stress was high during this time, setting the stage for the CVS to make its marked appearance.

Andrew, being highly intuitive, picked up on all these emotions and started to show more and more signs of struggling emotionally and physically. He began to have more and more trouble regulating energy and handling a lot of commotion and crowded places. While other kids would love to play a game of soccer, for Andrew it became his worst fear. For him there were too many unknowns and moving parts to process in a very short time. His body was showing more and more signs stress impacting him more than other kids his age and it was more than just anxiety. We still did not know how best to address this. We took him to Occupational Therapy for sensory integration issues hoping to help him respond in a more age-appropriate way to outside stimulation. We hoped to desensitize him to these things by placing him in preschool with an Individual Education Plan or IEP. Still things continued to get worse and worse.

In the fall of 2011, Andrew welcomed a new baby sister and began preschool, which was challenging for him as well. School was not the welcome break and time of fun we were hoping that it would be. We had hoped it would provide the consistency and predictability that he so desperately needed. Unfortunately it became a landmine of stressors. Doctors by this time were tossing around the question of whether he was on the autism spectrum because of his behaviors. It would take until 2014 before they would finally diagnosis him with autism in addition to the CVS.

I believe it was in March of 2011 that Andrew first went to the emergency room for a clear vomiting-related issue. He had been throwing up all night. It was the following daylight savings time, spring ahead, which is an often overlooked change that can trigger cycles. He was throwing up black tar-like goo, which was something new to us. My husband brought him in to the hospital for treatment this time. It was a scary sight, as the only time I had heard of such thing was on the popular medical show *House*, where medical mysteries are solved. Did our son warrant being on a show like this? How could this be? We were told it was just blood from the forceful retching that he had done. Little did I know that within a few months, even this would no longer faze me, as it would become a common occurrence. For a while the medications they gave us at the emergency room would be enough to control it. And then they stopped working.

While I was at the hospital with our youngest son who was having his tonsils out, I got the call from my husband, saying that Andrew was throwing up and did not seem able to stop, again. I was already exhausted from Greg's surgery, and I would then have to jump straight back into advocating for Andrew with no sleep. We had needed medical treatment for his cycles several times before at this point, so I knew (or so I thought but that was all about to change) what it would involve. I joked with the nurses, "Oh what, I am going to have two kids in here at the same time?" Well, I was almost correct. As I was arriving home with Greg, Dan headed off to the ER with Andrew.

However, this was not just a basic episode at all. This one would end with a full seven day admission and earn us an official diagnosis of CVS. We assumed that IV fluids and IV Zofran would be what stopped the cycle. We figured it would be like the last time—treat and release. When this did not happen, we entered a strange new journey in search of treatment plan that could control the vomiting. This would take about two years of numerous hospital admissions, medication trials, and several specialists to treat.

I started having vivid flashbacks to my childhood when I saw him just lying there in pain and unable to swallow even his own saliva. They gave him the Zofran, but this did very little, partially because he was unable to take it even with the dissolvable tablets. Even the IV version of the medication did very little to help. His pain was so unbearable he stopped talking and did not fight anyone who came to get blood work. This was clearly not my son, who was typically a handful when it came to cutting his fingernails or haircuts, let alone a needle. He was still retching blood and vomiting up to ten times an hour. This had been going on for twelve hours straight.

This time his pain was through the roof and his body kept contorting like a seizure. He grew paler and most of the color drained from his face. A code was called on him, meaning an emergency situation where any or every doctor in the area comes running into help. The team also called in a pulmonary team to investigate why he was doing this. When he was still contorting, the team decided he was hyperventilating after rushing lab work and giving him oxygen. They did not want to give him anything for the pain for fear it might mask a symptom that could lead to a diagnosis. So we sat there all night like this. I wanted to give them a chance to figure this out on their own (or until I could figure this out as it had been a part of my whole life).

During this time, I thought and thought. I knew there was a cycle pattern to this thing. What that meant and what it I was I didn't know. But I remembered watching the clock as a kid, just trying to go from throwing up every two minutes to five minutes to holding out for the ten minute goal. I knew what he felt like, and I felt helpless as to what to do to help him. This went on for five days. I searched the web for anything related to throwing up in cycles and, after some time, came across the Cyclic Vomiting Association web page and their treatment plan. I found Dr. David Fleischer's *Empirical Guidelines for Treating Cyclic Vomiting Syndrome*, which gave me something to use as I advocated for my son. Hope really does start there as their slogan claims.

I asked the hospitalist to try Zofran and Ativan. He said he was willing at that point to try it and was calling in a specialist as well. They called over the Pediatric GI doctor from Massachusetts General who worked at the specialty outreach clinic at the hospital (and the same doctor whom we had seen a few weeks before for constipation). He walked in and saw Andrew who was pale, drooling, and barely responsive. After asking me a few questions, he shared with us that this was a classic CVS textbook case. He himself had CVS as child and knew well what it looked like and how it felt. God sent us a specialist, who has since been a tremendous gift to our family.

We were able to see Boston's best without the stressful drive into the city. But more than that, he was someone who got it, who treated my son like a person and not a condition. At times, we found that some doctors treat children within the parameter of their specialty and fail to see the whole child. This time around we were able to find someone who did not do this. We also had a wonderful, compassionate pediatrician who was willing to learn and listen to our concerns. She called over and sent the nurses a packet of information on CVS for them to read. The hospital then chose a handful of nurses to learn about CVS and take over his care when he was admitted. They came to know his ins and outs and how to do what he needed. There were a few nurses who never got it, but after requesting those nurses not be assigned to him, we've never had a bad experience. His nurse Joette was fabulous, remembering that his favorite color was yellow and always seeking out that color of Popsicle when he was feeling well enough to have one.

For some, the diagnosis of Cyclic Vomiting Syndrome is overwhelming and unfamiliar. For me, it was a name to an enemy that plagued my childhood and made me fear vomiting. For me, to learn its name and that there was a plan was a huge relief. When I reflect back on receiving the diagnosis, it has been nothing but a blessing in my mind. We now know what we are dealing with, and more than that we have options to help him. For me, this is all that matters. We have medications that we can give him to try to reduce the severity and frequency of his episodes. We also know that, if all that fails, we can take him to the hospital for IV medications and fluids needed to ride out the cycle. This is huge progress compared to the lack of awareness

30 years ago. We are taking huge steps to a better quality of life for these kids.

CVS will most likely continue to be part of our kids' lives, and we can't change that. I cannot magically wish CVS away, though I'd like to. It's not very realistic. Instead, I will do the next best thing: I will learn everything there is to know about Cyclic Vomiting to become the best advocate possible for him. We will continue to seek out answers and better ways to help and minimize CVS's interruptions in our lives. Now there is hope.

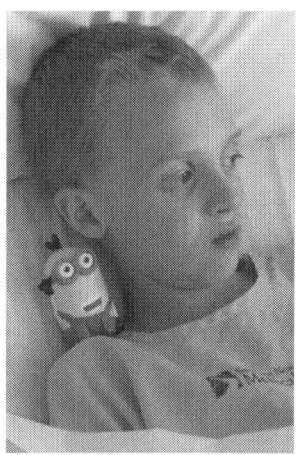
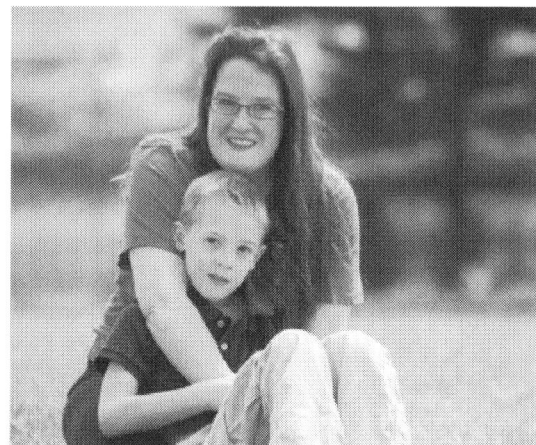

Ten Things CVS Children Wish Parents/ Caregivers Knew

There are things that CVS children wish their caregivers knew. Personally I've experienced both perspectives, having been a CVS kid as well as the parent of a CVS kid. My husband, on the other hand, had no prior experience with CVS. I have learned that there are some common mistakes made by those who haven't experienced CVS themselves. CVS is a whole different world with its own type of vomiting. Many well-intentioned parents make rookie mistakes. Here are some things your CVS kids wish they could tell you.

1. I don't do this on purpose. I get excited about birthdays, holidays, field trips and overnights. They sound like so much fun, but for some reason my body processes this excitement differently. The signal misfires and sets off a cycle. For some of us, hormones can also set it off. Whatever it is, I do not choose this.

2. I don't mean to miss the toilet. The need to vomit and the pain is so intense I can barely move, open my eyes, or even listen to your voice. So please forgive me if puking into a towel is the closest thing I can do. The mere thought of lifting my head is too much for me at times. Thank you for keeping a bucket near my bed and cleaning up my messes.

3. I wish I could swallow my own saliva. Between the taste of it mixing with bile and/or bloody mucus, I cannot do it. I'm terrified it will trigger more vomit since, well, everything does. Any sound, movement, touch, or breeze is too much for my nervous system. The one thing that would help the most is hydration. It is also, at the same time, the biggest aggravation to this cycle I am stuck in.

4. I may need IV fluid to get me through my episode. It's not because I don't want to swallow, it's that anything that goes down will come back up. Oral medications are the biggest joke if you are actually in a true Cyclic Vomiting cycle. They won't work. I may even ask for a suppository or even a shot to make this pain and cycle stop. Listen to me. Help me please.

5. I need a QUIET, DARK, Happy Place with NO MOVEMENT! We can name it whatever we like, my happy place, safe place, or battle ground. I may love a weighted blanket to comfort me, and possibly a white noise machine or fan pointed in another direction. Please don't wash me up right away, turn on lights, or talk to me to see how I'm feeling or flush the toilet near me. Any of those things will cause me to vomit so choose which you need to do wisely. Once I start vomiting, it is hard to stop. Please just stay nearby so I know you are there. I get scared and feel like

I'm dying and might faint. Actually, I might wish I'd faint as that would mean less pain for a short time.

6. I'm hot, then I'm cold. As the urge to puke gets more intense I get hot, blotchy and sweaty. I may throw off covers suddenly. After I throw up, I tend to get the chills and shake. This repeats over and over again. Don't put a lot of clothes on me to keep me warm. Just a blanket will do. After I throw up, I feel the best I'm going to feel until the episode is over so only ask me questions at that time. Otherwise, I'm too busy trying not to throw up and don't have the energy to answer you. I am busy riding out the storm.

7. I love you! I hate this just as much as you do. Thank you for helping me through this. Thank you for seeking treatment when I needed it. Thank you for not seeing this as a failure or the result of either of us not trying hard enough. It's just the nature of CVS. We will figure this out together. I know you are there to help me. Listen to me when I talk, and I promise to do my best to do as you ask.

8. You are my rock. No matter how bad I look, quietly cheer me on. When you freak out, I freak out. So stay calm and then you can freak out later. Take advantage of online support groups so that you don't feel so alone. We may not know too many people near us that have this battle, so seek people out. It will help all of us feel more normal and validated.

9. If school is too much for me, that's ok. This is not a failure. It's just an alternative lifestyle. There's never been a better time for home-schooling since Internet programs, charter schools and co-ops are on the rise in the United States. With so many parents opting for this, we are hardly alone. It need not be just a curse of CVS; it could also be a blessing of it. For more information, search "hack schooling" on the Internet. It's amazing! Just look at what this home school kid does. This could be me! Together we can do this!

10. And remember, cycles do not happen all the time (typically), and no matter how many hospital admissions we have that

complicate family events and holidays, we still have a good life. Our life looks different than others, but I would not change it. I also don't know it any other way. To me this is normal.

An Otherwise "Typical" Childhood Interrupted by CVS

Childhood is often thought of as a special and carefree time where we make our first impressions of the world around us. It's a time of building snow forts, playing in the rain, building sandcastles and riding bikes until the sun goes down. It is during this time we learn to do basic things such as walk, talk, play with others, and eventually to read and write. It's a period of self-discovery and exploration, where the only job you have is to play and learn. It is this time that a child should feel safe and secure. If childhood prepares kids for the future, what does the future hold for CVS kids?

A child with CVS can often appear to be like other children their same age, until they begin to throw up. Every child from time to time gets sick and vomits because they have a virus or they ate too much. Some throw up when they are nervous and then feel better. Our CVS children commonly vomit six times or more per hour for hours on end. They are frequently ill on holidays, birthdays and vacation any time that would otherwise bring a child joy. Marie Healy, a fellow CVS mom, described CVS as being a condition that is "the biggest bully. When you're happy, it's there to get you. When you're scared, it's there to get you. You just can't catch a break." It's definitely not your typical vomiting, as you will learn how it often differs in the frequency and intensity.

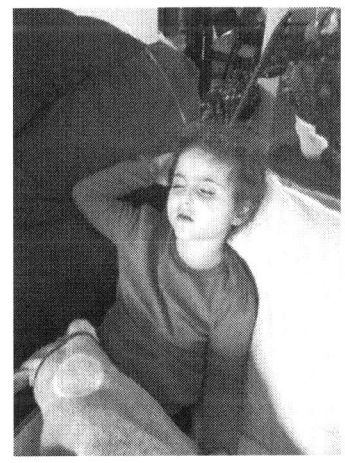

For some kids, CVS only makes an occasional appearance 3-4 times a year and lasts for only a day or so. Others, however, are not so lucky and cycle 12 or more times per year, often requiring hospitalizations. The pattern can vary year to year as the child grows. Some years can be good while others can be traumatic and difficult to get through. Much depends on what the child's triggers are and how they are managed. CVS can be very unpredictable and therefore challenging to manage.

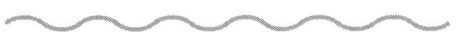

My Life Every 12-1/2 Weeks

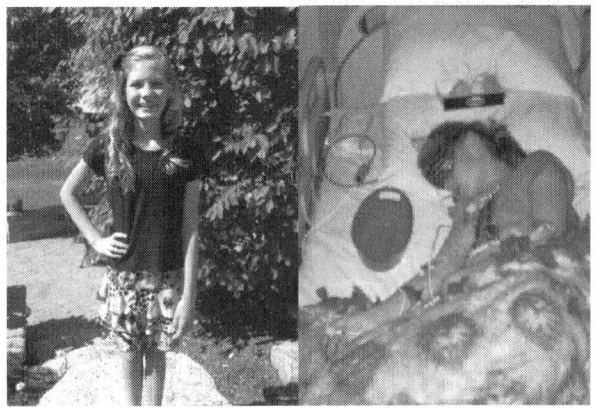

Julia Benway

Just another episode….Not being able to do anything for days and days. I can't even open my eyes, move or talk! I am in the hospital with an IV getting lots of fluids and medicines. I don't remember hardly anything. So DIZZY! I can't even explain, words cannot express how I feel when I have CVS. My ribs are sore from throwing up. I am missing school, parties, hanging out with my friends, gymnastics and much more. The light and noise KILLS. Nobody can understand CVS, but me and other sufferers. The pain I go through every 12-1/2 weeks is deadly. Sometimes I feel very alone.

I am 14 years old and have been suffering from CVS since the age of 4. I am hopeful that one day I will grow out of this illness and that doctors will find a cure for Cyclic Vomiting Syndrome.

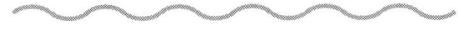

Some physicians dismiss the vomiting as a phase or a virus. Some will say it is just something the child has to outgrow, even if they give the proper diagnosis of CVS. Since CVS is considered a self-limited condition, some parents and doctors feel it's best to let it ride its course, leaving the child to suffer through the cycle for days. A self-limited condition is one that resolves on its own with or without treatment. For other children, cycles mean hospital trips complete with numerous tests that often leave the doctors and parents with more questions than answers and expensive medical bills. The ones who are blessed go on to receive a treatment plan, which often includes medications to prevent future episodes and advice on how to support the child at the onset of an episode. Valera Leigh Hilt, a CVS mother from Nevada, USA, shares her experience:

> Since then, he has had countless medical tests and procedures. Now even as these have settled down and we have a steady protocol to follow when he goes into an episode, he still really hates the hospital and IVs and taking meds. Who wouldn't? I try so hard to keep CVS from robbing him of his childhood and his innocence.

No matter what your child's treatment plan or diagnosis status, children with CVS quickly learn their limitations. Having Cyclic Vomiting Syndrome does shape the childhood of those who have it, often setting children who have it apart from their peers. Patrick (age 8) of Colorado describes that feeling of separation:

> CVS changes everything about how you live: needing more sleep, needing to eat more regularly, needing to rest and have quiet time (even as an older kid). It's hard to keep up with all the things I want to do; it's hard to feel good and be happy. I feel bad that I have CVS, and I often wonder why no one can figure out how to help me.

Tayarra Smith, a teen from New South Wales, Australia, has struggled with CVS and other health issues for the last two years. She became ill so frequently that her mother chose to enroll her in a distance education program so that she could keep up with schoolwork. She shared her feelings about living with CVS:

> Sometimes you have to stop yourself from crying because you are stronger than that. Other times you have to cry. It's because you've been strong for too long. But while you are crying you have to think positive. It is hard. All of your friends are going to birthdays, partying, etc. And you get invited but you have to say no to them. They understand and they cancel their plans and come over to my house. Sometimes I don't want them to come because my pain is so severe (my pain tolerance is high now), my skin is pale yellowish and you just look so sick. They could see I have lost a lot of weight. It's not easy going through stomach issues. But you know you are going to get through it with your friends and family. With the medical stuff, surgeons, etc. They are so supportive. They become like my family... I know it's weird but they feel like family. Especially the nurses in emergency, etc. But I'm used to it.

This illness affects more than just the child; it affects everyone around them including parents, siblings, friends, and teachers. It can often keep families on edge, never knowing what to expect. Kyra's parents share the impact that CVS has on their lives:

> Our world stops with that first vomit. We go to hospital never knowing whether the doctor or nurses we see will even know about CVS. The same questions, the hours in delay, till they put the drip line (IV fluids) and meds in. No matter that we carry our own paper work from a specialist that works at the same hospital...my daughter suffers terrible stomach pain nearly all the time now but there are no answers for this.....the only

upside is that with age and daily meds the episodes are now less frequent 4-5 months. Duration is two days once drip line and meds are in and recovery about four days.

From any early age CVS leaves a lasting impression on our kids. The older they get, the more they are able to express what it feels like to them. When they are young we might see its impacts on their behavior as many become anxious and withdrawn at times. There are kids who also display obsessive compulsive behaviors in attempts to have control over something after having been so weak and vulnerable during episodes. Some are able to verbalize it, while others are able to show you by what they create or do when they play. They do have an opinion on the subject and it's important to acknowledge these thoughts. Some kids will act out in aggression or anger, or feel scared. It's important to help them with these feelings.

Some children take to creative means such as drawing, writing, Legos or Minecraft to work through the emotions that go along with cyclic vomiting. Some decorate puke buckets like Katie.

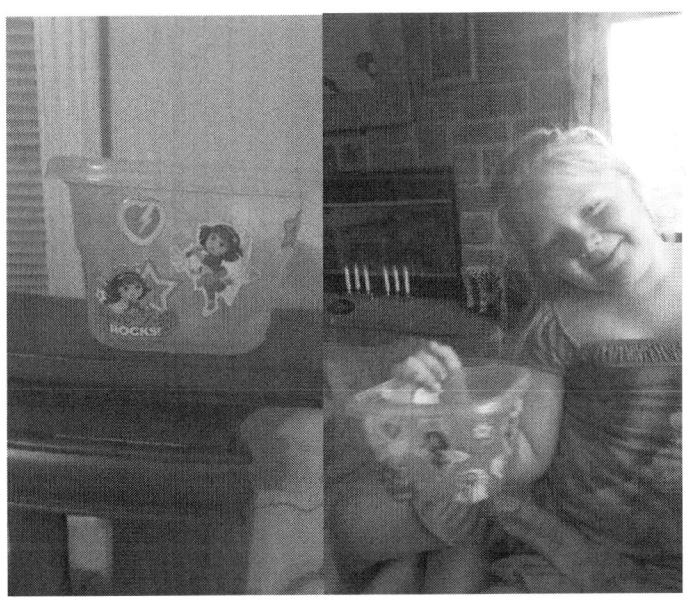

Below is a Lego model my son made after repeated hospital stays. For him, it became normal to go there, and CVS became a normal topic of his free play. While other kids he knew were off at soccer games and birthday parties, he spent most of the last two years in the hospital praying that something, anything, might break the wave of a cycle that is repeatedly making him painfully vomit for hours on end.

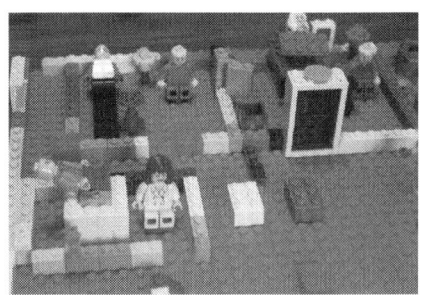 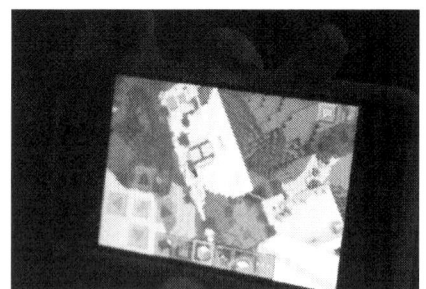

Jenny Owens shares a similar story:

My son came home from the last day of school today with another abdominal migraine and severe diarrhea. When this happens we have found that if we let him play video games in a dark quiet room it helps take his mind off it for a while. While watching him play Minecraft I realized that EVERY world he has designed and built has a hospital and "doctor" character in it. At first it made me kind of sad that this is his reality, but I asked him why he did that. He said he couldn't imagine living in a world where you couldn't go get some help and medicines, so he didn't want anyone else to have to either. Our kids may go through way more pain and sickness than children should have to, but they definitely come out of it with a lot of compassion and empathy. Who knows? Maybe one of our kids or one of us will be the one to comes up with an answer and really effective treatment so these kids don't have to suffer in the future!

Many CVS kids have had thoughts, or even spoken out loud, of wanting to die. Typically, they are not actually suicidal, just scared and overwhelmed by the pain. Personally, I remember feeling conflicted both with a great fear of fainting and welcoming it. It's easy as an onlooker to say these kids are okay and suggest they "ride it out at home" and not seek medical treatment. Many doctors tell parents to watch for extreme signs of dehydration. Severe dehydration, however, should not be the only reason to seek treatment. The intense pain, weakness and sheer frequency of vomiting should also be considered in the decision of when treatment is provided. This level of pain can have an impact on the mental health of our children. It's easy to see why they would develop anxiety about getting sick.

I do not like when I throw up. It is gross. Feels like a nasty taste. It burns my throat. ...Cause the throw up helps me get the air out. When my belly hurts, it tells me when to throw up. I go to the IV hospital. I like the hospital but I do not like IVs.

— Hope, age 4

Tiffany Sharpe (of Trinity's Troops) and her five year old daughter Trinity wrote this poem to try to explain to others what CVS feels like.

When I get the pukies it feels pretty yucky.
Then I get the feeling I'm not so lucky.
I have to lay down and be quiet and still.
Then my mommy will give me a pill.
Sometimes it lasts for quite a few hours,
When all I want to do is go pick some flowers.
I always get the pukies on the worst days.
When all of my friends can go out and play.
Sometimes I have to go to the hospital to help me get strong.
Then when I'm all better I can sing lots of songs.
God made me this way and that's all I can be.
I know that Jesus will never forget about me.

Sometimes it makes my mommy very sad.
I just want to get better to make her happy and glad.
I love my mommy and daddy and they really try,
I pray that one day the pukies will go bye, bye.

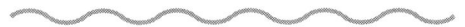

Often I think the words the children use to describe how it feels make for a better description than you would find in any medical journal. The kids speak in simple ways that can help one to easily imagine what the pain must be like. Thomas, age 7, describes how he "hates it when I am sick and vomit. My head feels like a volcano," he says. Patrick, age 8, describes how CVS "sucks the energy out of my body and spirit. It keeps me from playing sports the way I know I can, from playing with my friends as much as I want, and makes me feel bad about who I am." Some, such as Natalie, age 9, express that on occasion they felt so bad that they thought they were going to die. Brianna, one of the older kids I spoke with, shared how she starts "vomiting every 35-40 minutes for eight hours or more. I vomit bile and often have the taste of blood when I vomit. It makes me weak and dehydrated. The following day I really don't feel like eating much and my stomach is also very sore."

Our children have to deal with more health issues than regular stomach viruses and colds. As a result, CVS kids can experience a lot of anxiety. Pamela Souter shares her son's experiences: "This disease is causing him much anxiety as he matures, and he is becoming increasingly apprehensive—not knowing when it will strike again." His fear of when will it hit again will often aggravate the condition and increase the likelihood that it will happen again. What's key, as you will see, is providing creative and safe ways for children to work through these fears. Some are able to talk about it, others share in other ways. There are many unknowns that often go along with having CVS. When will the next episode hit? Will I be able to get the medical treatment I need? How long will I be sick this time? As a result of these uncertainties, they take nothing for granted.

You will read later about the successes of these kids and their families. It is our job as parents to help them get there. So never give up hope. These children are amazingly strong. They can live a good life even with CVS when they have parents who are willing to support them. In conclusion, our children's non-adherence to vomit standards are the result of a known medical condition and not poor parenting or a mental condition.

No child with CVS freely or intentionally chooses to vomit that much, nor can they control it once it is set in motion. It's similar to a tornado forming: once in motion, it takes on a life of its own. A non-CVS child with the stomach flu would be the equivalent to a windy day, whereas a CVS cycle would be like an F5 Tornado. The difference is the intensity. While all children get sick and throw up from time to time, CVS should be viewed differently and be treated differently. Sadly, too many children are written off as just as having the flu, time and time again, or being told they are anxious or making themselves sick. Thankfully, more and more awareness is being raised in the general population and in the medical community.

Unique Behaviors of Children During a Cycle

For years I had thought of myself as weak, or odd, or challenging for the odd behaviors I would have when I was sick, throwing up in the mid-1980s. My older brother did not throw up like this. No one else in my family did, nor did anyone else we knew. So you can imagine my surprise when I saw my son responding in the exact same ways as I remembered doing as a child. He would barely be able to move or even lift his head to throw up let alone have any thought of reaching the toilet. I felt a huge wave of validation come over me as I read more and more stories of other children exhibiting these behaviors. There was more to it though. It was not only that they did similar things, but these things were actually hallmarks of the condition of which we were unaware.

Unless you have witnessed a cycle yourself firsthand, it is easy to believe that the person is grossly exaggerating. During the early months I kept a log of the times he threw up and noted the exact pattern every cycle took. This pattern stayed the same until we were able to find the right combination of meds to shut it down fully.

Andrew would wake up and vomit at 5:35 in the morning. And then at 5:45. And at 6:00, 6:12, 6:20, 6:30, 6:45, 6:59, 7:19, 7:36, 7:50, 8:10, and 8:30. Yes, you read that correctly. Within the first three hours of the cycle he had thrown up thirteen times! And the vomiting only continued. Around 10:30 am we brought him to the emergency room, and were able to be admitted and in a pediatric room by 2:00 pm, at which time I stopped my official count of times he vomited. He was now in a quiet dark room with his panda eye mask on and his starry night weighted blanket that I made for him. Once in the room he would attempt to watch TV but have to turn it off because it was too much stimulation and he would vomit all over again. He is often bothered by any sound, even people talking. He's also sensitive to light, being touched, and having to move. He does not talk during these episodes, and tends only to use hand motions. When his siblings came to visit the next day, he began to vomit all over again because of the stimulation. So we would keep visitors away and try to ride it out in our quiet dark "bat cave" or "happy place."

They were giving him Ativan and Zofran along with IV fluids, which took away some of the pain and somewhat diminished the frequency of retching. At 3:30 pm the following day, a full 30 hours after the onset, he entered what we have termed the *chipmunk phase*. During this phase he will not talk or swallow his own salvia. He puffs out his cheeks as they fill with salvia. He will do this until the pain is gone. I've seen this time and time again. At this point it has been hours since he last actively vomited and nursing staff think he is better. They do not see that the cycle is still in progress. It appears that he was spitting and not swallowing on purpose, yet no bribes or punishments are able to change his behavior. It is not until 6:00 the following morning that the on/off switch gets flipped.

Many CVS kids have what I would like to call the *on/off switch* end to the cycles. To my surprise, I am not the only one to have called it that. Dr. Li, from Children's Hospital of Wisconsin, also described it as a signature "on/off" pattern. This type of ending is abrupt. One minute they are in conscious coma barely responding (typically after deep sleep) and the next they are waking up and asking for bacon, and they are able to eat it. We have learned that when an episode is in progress there is nothing we can do to alter its course other than sleep, and when it's over, it's over. Just like that.

> And then 45 minutes after throwing up, she sat up in bed, declared her teddy smelled of puke, and 25 minutes after that, she is eating, drinking, watching TV, has put her clothes on, brushed her teeth and hair and pulled out a loose tooth.
>
> It never stops amazing me: from conscious coma to completely normal within minutes. When she was four she started an episode (undiagnosed at the time), lasting from the 22nd of December until the afternoon of the 26th, when she sat up and demanded her presents and Christmas dinner.
>
> —Elin from Norway, discussing her 8-year-old daughter.

Today among many child psychologists and educators there is a philosophy that if a child could, he or she would. However, too many others are quick to suggest that willfulness is the cause of the unique behavior. We need to make sure that people who are treating our children understand that if they could stop vomiting, they would. I have experienced only setbacks when nursing staff are instructed to force him to eat or drink. They would take away TV and games and such to use as incentives or to motivate him which actually creates more stress and anxiety and starts the whole cycle over again.

In my experience it is typically best to wait until the switch is flipped off before offering any food or beverage. The typical protocol of even introducing food slowly does not tend to be true for us. If they can they will drink or eat. We have found often that my son could go from eating nothing for two days or more and then was able to transition to a desired food such as bacon immediately without problems. How is this possible? Because the switch has been flipped and normal messages are being sent to the stomach about how to behave.

If these cycles were a just a stomach virus, it might be different. The stomach might benefit from gradual introduction of bland food and progress slowly. An informational pamphlet created by the Cyclical Vomiting Association of the UK makes note of this approach as being the one that nurses and hospital staff should take with CVS patients. They believe that "all patients will begin to talk, drink and take care of themselves when the nausea recedes and they feel well again. It may be better to let the patient determine the pace" (CVSUK, Nursing Patients with CVS).

> I clearly remember in one episode of CVS, my daughter all of the sudden asking for crackers. I always take them to the hospital with us to munch on. I was hesitant, but gave the box to my little one. She ate 24 crackers and her episode was over. The ironic thing about it is she is mostly reliant on her tube for nutrition so I was ecstatic about her eating them.
>
> — Melissa Knight

Nursing patients with CVS, from the Cyclical Vomiting Association United Kingdom, documents many of the challenging or odd behaviors[1]:

- *Hypersalivation, drooling, refusal to swallow*
  Swallowing, even saliva, can cause gagging, retching and an increase in nausea. Patients may dribble or spit, or hold their saliva in their mouths (inhibiting speech). They may refuse to swallow water or oral medications.
- *Unusual posture*
  Because of severe abdominal pain, patients may adopt unusual postures. They may be reluctant to move as movement intensifies nausea.

---

[1] http://www.cvsa.org.uk/downloads/leaflets/204%20Nursing%20leaflet.pdf

- *Withdrawal- Conscious Coma*
  Intense, intractable nausea and exhaustion can lead to total withdrawal. Patients may show no interest in their surroundings and may be unwilling to talk, read or watch TV. Children may refuse to take part in school or play activities. Alternatively patients may become tearful, irritable, rude or demanding.
- *Compulsive water drinking*
  Patients may attempt to alleviate retching by drinking large amounts of water. Water also dilutes the acidity of the vomit and thereby reduces the burning sensation in the esophagus when vomiting. It is futile to try to stop this behavior as this only increases the patient's distress.

Melissa Knight shared the following with me: "If it were not for your post or blog about kids needing to spit and not swallow, I would have panicked. Last night she couldn't sleep. She kept spitting in a towel constantly, every drop of saliva in her mouth she spat out and she was rubbing the towel on her tongue and using her fingers to get rid of any remaining saliva. If you hadn't written that I would've called the doctor because it looked odd and obsessive, so thanks!"

While we may not be any kind of medical expert, we are the experts on our children. We know our children best. We are a key piece for helping the doctors and nursing staff in providing care for our kids. We know what is normal for them and what is not. We also become experts on what qualifies as "normal" cycle behavior. The professionals are in charge of many kids over the course of the day. Every child is different and the teams make generalizations as part of the job. It is for this reason that we need to speak up for our children and help their nursing staff to understand them and the particularities of their cyclic vomiting syndrome.

The behaviors mentioned above are just some of the unique coping skills that our cyclic vomiting kids develop over time. Many of these children are willing to tell us when it is time to head to the hospital, and some do as early as age four. They have been known to beg for an IV or suppository with full knowledge of what it means. By outside standards this might seem crazy, but to them it is the only chance to get some relief from the crippling spasms and retching that their body is engaging in.

So many of our kids rejoice once they have progressed from vomiting every five minutes to vomiting every ten minutes and then to every 30 minutes. They often learn to set simple goals during cycles, such being able to swallow their own saliva before taking sips of other liquids. I also use the trick of setting the goal to get my son to talk to me, which then results with him swallowing automatically without thinking. Sometimes children cannot swallow out of fear. Others seem to have forgotten how. They have to learn from experience when they can tolerate oral liquid and when they cannot. And they do. It's a tough balance between fear and pain.

They may have had the experience of overhearing a doctor telling us that they look like they were in a concentration camp, after a mere 24 hours at home trying to abort a cycle. Many of them have often been in the emergency room so often that the staff almost rolls out the red carpet. It's not every patient that can tell you what gauge needle to use and where to best place the IV. The nursing staff often loves us because we are very self-sufficient; we know where the nurses keep the linen and things, and we freely get what we need. CVS caregivers and CVS kids are a rare breed indeed. We share many of the above mentioned common traits that just appear odd to outsiders. They may be odd behaviors but are all a normal part of living with Cyclic Vomiting Syndrome.

Invisible Illness

From the outside CVS often seems to be an invisible illness because there are no tests to document that it is occurring other than direct observations and lack of known cause. It's also difficult to identify because of its on/off switch phenomena, which is mistaken as being within the child's control. The periods of wellness in between can make people doubt that the condition is anything more than a way of seeking attention or a mental condition. Many parents have to encounter accusations of faking it on a daily basis.

> "From the time Caleb was three I've had people tell me he is faking it. They thought that I love having this attention on him and that I am making this illness up. I've had doctors tell me there was nothing they or I could do for him.
>
> My son did get help! We found a doctor willing to hear me. We treated the symptoms, yes, but by doing so we are almost a year vomit free… Caleb wasn't making this happen to himself. I did not like seeing him suffer or make this up!!!! CVS is real! And don't let anyone tell you differently!"
>
> —Lori Kenison

Some CVS children have suffered greatly from misguided staff, one such child to the point of being placed in a mental facilities. Kristina Kruse has such a story and shared how she was treated at the tender age of 10. She describes how the "nurses there locked me into a small padded blue room and told me, 'Until you get out of the behavior, you are staying in here.' After four and a half hours I was eventually let out, but it was not before I had puked and had a bowel movement all over myself." Thankfully Kristina's mother was allowed to discharge her daughter and seek care elsewhere.

It my the hope that the information presented here will be read by medical professionals, nurses, and families who will then be able to see what CVS really is and how it is experienced by those who have first-hand experience caring for those who suffer with it. It is not meant to be formal or official research, but rather a survey of experiences set out before the world to say that we are worth helping. We are worth the time and money for the wider medical community to pay attention to us. As a community, we are still fairly new; however, we have come so far in a short time. It is only a matter of time before we are able to offer future CVSers even more hope.

Cycle Pattern and Cycle Frequency

Often the term cycle is used in two ways when discussing cyclic vomiting syndrome, cycle pattern, and cycle frequency. *Cycle pattern* refers to the stages of vomiting that a child goes through. For example, a cycle pattern might involve a child waking up at 3:00 am, throwing up every five minutes for the first hour, and then by 6:00 am the vomiting slows to every 15 minutes, after which the child enters a conscious coma phase, before returning to normal after sleeping five hours. This pattern can vary from person to person, but each person tends to have his or her own predictable pattern. These patterns stay the same unless an effective intervention can be found and used to abort or stop the process.

Cycle frequency refers to the length of time between the start of one cycle and the start of the next one. For some kids it varies because of stressors. Other kids are known as "calendar kids" who cycle every certain number of days. What marks the end of one cycle and the start of the next is the return to a symptom free phase between the cycles. In some cases, kids have such a short symptom free phase that it is difficult to tell when one cycle ends and the next begins. In our experience, we call this the "yo-yo phase." For example, our son would seemingly be better, sit up and eat, and then 30 minutes later he would go back into a full cycle. One time we were about to be discharged, and right before they removed the IV he started vomiting again, which resulted in the addition of another day to our hospital stay. Others refer to this phase as rapid cycling, or coalescence (which means to grow together), where the lines overlap and become blurred.

> She went into this period where episodes overlapped so one began before the other ended AND she didn't always vomit but had 10 out of 10 nausea and couldn't move. This went on for months.
>
> — Nicole Dion

In Adam's case we have had both where we have cycled with maybe a day or two or a few hours (12-24) of wellness in between cycles. Usually he is admitted when we are unable to treat at home. They use the drug DHE on Adam to try to break the cycle on him, along with Reglan, Zofran and Ativan. Plus he takes his normal "preventatives."

This is when he usually hits rock bottom emotionally. This rapid cycling really wears on him and, well, all of us! I think all I can say is don't try to tough it out at home for too long; go in for help. It really does help. I have a strong support system of friends, the CVS Moms' group, family and great doctors, all of which helps so much. If we didn't have great doctor and hospital I don't know what we would do!

— Kimberly Bell

Children with CVS tend to fall into one of the two categories trigger kids and calendar kids. There are those children who have triggers that can be identified and those whose cycle occur every certain number of days like clockwork, who are commonly referred to as calendar kids. The harder to treat of the two categories are the calendar kids, because there is nothing that can be avoided to prevent the cycle. More studies need to be done to better understand these different types of cyclic vomiting syndrome, as well as to better understand the age of onset.

These unique and often misunderstood behaviors our children display during a cycle can be very overwhelming and confusing to onlookers. Those around us may look at us and our children wondering what the heck is wrong with us, and now we can tell them we are dealing with an actual medical condition. We need to remember that these oddities are all part of living with a child with CVS. Take comfort in the fact that others are going through similar struggles as your child. We've come a long way in properly diagnosing CVS with the clearly defined criteria, and are still searching for effective treatments based on each child's particular triggers.

What is CVS: Mental Disorder or Medical Issue?

In my research and speaking with many families affected by CVS, I've discovered that there is still much that is unknown. Some of us have been told, "Oh it's just an anxiety disorder" or "It's just a food allergy." CVS, I've decided, is the unique way the body responds when it is presented with certain triggers. Other people have anxiety disorders and do not throw up in this way—because they do not have Cyclic Vomiting Syndrome. Most doctors agree that CVS is a neurologic disorder, at the present time it is believed to be related to a migraine variant. There are many different ways that the disorder can be triggered such as inner ear problems, undiagnosed food allergies, anxiety disorders and mitochondrial disease. It will take more in-depth studies and research to better formulate an official definition. While the medical community sort this out, we need to find ways to help our child day to day live with the condition as we seek out answers.

The Many Paths to a Diagnosis

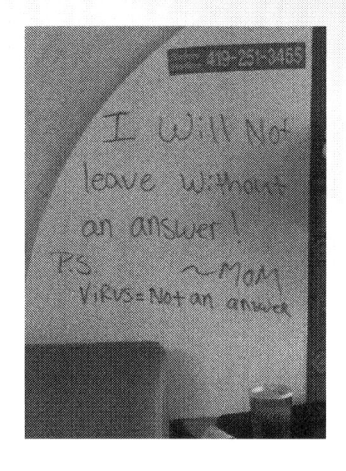

Each CVS family has a unique story to tell. We each arrive at a diagnosis differently. For some it takes years, for others months. We have sought medical treatment from a variety of providers hoping to find an answer. We have gone through a battery of testing such as MRI, CT scans, endoscopies, barium swallows, and many others. We've kept logs, and shared family histories, documented cycles in photos so others might believe us. As I shared easily it was a relatively quick diagnosis for my son, while I myself went totally undiagnosed. I found it very helpful to read others' experiences as I gathered them for this book.

The three main criteria included are:

- Recurrent, severe episodes of vomiting greater than six times an hour
- Normal health in between episodes
- No cause of vomiting found on testing

The four supportive criteria included:

- Each episode is similar to the other episodes
- Episodes resolve if they are left untreated (self-limited)
- Associated symptoms of nausea, abdominal pain, headache, motion sickness, and sensitivity to lights
- Associated signs of fever, paleness, diarrhea, dehydration, and excess salivation

There is no single test that is a definitive marker of CVS. It is a diagnosis of exclusion, meaning that the diagnosis is made when other causes of the vomiting have been ruled out, as well as by considering symptom history and family history. Each of us arrives at the diagnosis by different paths. There are many factors that impact how and when the diagnosis comes. If it is after the publication of the guidelines in 2008, it is much easier to receive. However it still depends on how experienced the medical team is in dealing with CVS.

Mollie's Path: Finding a Plan and Sharing with the World
Kathleen Adams, B.S.N., R.N Founder of Cyclic Vomiting Syndrome Association

My daughter, Mollie, was born in 1978 on her sister's sixth birthday after a happy, uneventful pregnancy. Her four-year-old brother was ready for another sister and her red-headed, freckled-faced presence filled our house with joy. At approximately age 12 months, Mollie was diagnosed with mild unidentified global developmental delays. When Mollie was about one and a half, she woke up one morning vomiting for no apparent reason. This was the beginning of eleven years of vomiting episodes that were mysterious, horrible, and undiagnosed.

Initially she vomited about two times, went to sleep for about two hours and then woke up her usual vigorous self. Six months later, this scene was repeated. About every six weeks for the next six months she did the same thing, but each episode of vomiting became a bit more extended. By the time she was about three years old she was having episodes about once a month or so, lasting for one to two days. In spite of multiple medical interventions for diagnosis and treatment, the cause of vomiting could not be determined and no suitable treatment was found.

During the years when Mollie was about four until she was about ten, she was admitted to the local children's hospital about every four to six weeks for IV therapy. The episodes lasted for two to four days. The nausea and vomiting were relentless. She would vomit about six to eight times an hour continuously except for some periods of sleep in between. She missed a great deal of school and the medical treatment needed was rigorous and left Mollie and our family in a wake of upheaval and deep distress.

In order to avoid the disruption of hospitalization, Mollie had central IV lines placed for home IV care over a period of about four years. Mollie's medical support team searched for answers about cause and treatment as relentlessly as she was vomiting. Nothing was found, and we continued to feel like we were the only family in the world with a child suffering from this miserable and mysterious illness.

Eleven years later, in 1990, by chance, our pediatrician found a letter to the editor in a medical journal describing a similar case. This letter led us to Dr. David Fleisher, MD, a pediatric gastroenterologist from the University of Missouri, Columbia. With Dr. Fleisher's immediate assessment and treatment plan, Mollie's condition began to improve at about the age of 13. Dr. Fleisher prescribed amitriptyline for Mollie at that time, which brought improvement in the frequency, duration and intensity of the episodes. Mollie continues to take amitriptyline today. During late adolescence the vomiting episodes transformed into migraine headaches. She suffered from migraines which started abating in her late 20s. Today, at the age of 35, she is essentially episode free with the exception of very short episodes of headache and/or vomiting triggered by anxiety or airline turbulence. Needless to say her life is much improved.

In 1999, Mollie was diagnosed via mitochondrial DNA samples with probable mitochondrial disease by a clinician and investigator doing studies about the relationship of CVS and mitochondrial disease. This diagnosis accounts for her mild cognitive disability.

In 1993, a handful of families from the USA and the United Kingdom came together in Milwaukee, Wisconsin for a weekend of comparing stories and making plans. Dr. Fleisher and Dr. B U.K. Li were present as well. Everyone gathered agreed to start CVSA – a medical non-profit. With the help of a strong and committed medical advisory team and some very dedicated patients, parents, and grandparents, there are now six CVS Associations around the globe and contact physicians and/or families in approximately 30 countries throughout the world. The global mission is one of outreach, education and research support. The Cyclic Vomiting Syndrome Association USA/Canada is at work in North America to find families still suffering in isolation and to promote and fund medical research to continue the search for answers about this devastating illness.

Of special note, it is not unheard of to have Social Services called in situations like Mollie's in order to rule out cases of Munchausen's Syndrome by Proxy. Ruling out this diagnosis is extremely important and relatively simple because of the unique symptomatology involved. The volunteers of CVSA are moving ahead with dogged determination to continue our outreach efforts to alert the medical community about CVS in order to prevent further unnecessary suffering in families that are already devastated by the effects of this illness.

Caitlin's Path: Building the Team for Hope Starts Here
Caitlin Baran

My journey with Cyclic Vomiting Syndrome started on January 25, 1987 (a little less than four months shy of my 4th birthday). While most families in the United States of America were watching the Giants defeat the Broncos in Super Bowl XXI, my mother and I were in the emergency room at the local hospital waiting for me to be seen by the newest pediatrician in the practice. I came down with what seemed like a stomach bug, except I continued to vomit to the point of dehydration. The pediatrician on call diagnosed me with a stomach bug, ordered IV fluids, and sent my mother and me on our merry way.

Little did we know this event would change the life of our family forever. These (stomach bug like) vomiting episodes would recur six to eight times a year over the course of the next six years. Each of these vomiting episodes equated to an admission to the hospital for roughly five days. I was taken to other hospitals in the state of PA several times during these mysterious instances of vomiting for days on end. This was so I could undergo testing (x-rays, CT scans, EEGs, and MRIs), and be seen by specialists. Unfortunately the testing didn't reveal anything and neither the specialists nor my pediatricians were any closer to figuring out what was causing these recurrent episodes of intense vomiting. Throughout this time I was prescribed various daily medications (anti-seizure medications, anti-anxiety medications, anti-migraine medications, and anti-nausea/vomiting medications); however, none of the medications stopped these still very mysterious episodes of vomiting from recurring.

One evening, when I was eight years old, my mother was reading Readers Digest when she came across information about the National Organization for Rare Diseases (NORD). This was the answer we had been waiting for over the past five years. NORD put my mother in touch with the President of the Cyclic Vomiting Syndrome Association (which at the time was just in its infancy). My parents and I were so glad to finally have a name for these inexplicable vomiting episodes. Not long after this, my parents traveled to Milwaukee, WI to meet with a small group which consisted of the President and founders of the Cyclic Vomiting Syndrome Association (CVSA), doctors who were on the cutting edge of Cyclic Vomiting Syndrome (CVS), other parents of children and adults with CVS, and several adults with CVS. It was at this meeting that my parents gathered some valuable information on CVS, including a protocol for what to do when I had an episode (which included being admitted to the hospital as soon as possible for IV fluids), ways to provide some relief during an episode (taking hot baths), and suggestions on eliminating these episodes completely (following an adaptive macrobiotic diet after coming out of the episode).

I began to follow an adaptive macrobiotic diet once my next episode was over. This meant avoiding foods containing dairy, sugar, wheat, preservatives, and fried foods. Basically when my episode was over all I was permitted to eat was rice, very well cooked vegetables, beef or poultry, and some fruits. The reasoning behind this diet was to give my body a chance to heal. After I started following the adaptive macrobiotic diet my episodes gradually began to decrease. Also, slowly, over the course of many years I was able to add more foods in. Coincidence or not, I am proud to say that I have been episode free for 14 years and counting.

Irelynn's Path: Googling
Brianne Hannigan

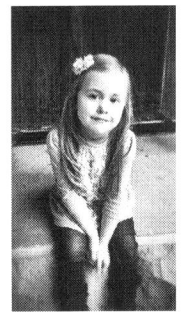

Irelynn's first episode started about year and a half ago, right after she turned three. One night she woke up throwing up over and over again and I thought, *Great! The flu has hit our house!* Then the next morning she woke up like nothing happened. This continued, on and off, sometimes on a daily basis, for about eight months, and none of our other three kids ever caught the flu. I would start to get nervous that maybe something was wrong with her, but then a few weeks would go by and she would seem fine, and I would kind of put it in the back of my mind, just hoping that maybe she did just catch viruses easier.

One night after one of her episodes started I decided to start googling. I typed in, why does my child throw up at the same time every night (because that was what I found to be the weirdest part of it all), and up popped CVS. I started reading and it was like someone had wrote about exactly what I had been living for the last year.

The next day I made an appointment with her pediatrician. I told him about what was going on and my thoughts as to what it could be. He didn't think it could be CVS because it wasn't severe enough but referred her to a pediatric GI anyways. We are very lucky that her GI doctor listened to my story and immediately told me he thought it was CVS. It still took a few months from that point to get the final diagnoses of CVS because of all of the testing she had to go through first. She was finally diagnosed last February, so we are still new to this CVS journey and have a lot to learn. So far we started her on COQ10 and L-Carnitine every day, and Zofran and Benadryl once an episode starts.

After sitting here thinking back on her life we did have warning signs that something was not normal with her as early as six months old. During her first Christmas Eve family gathering, she started violently vomiting over and over. It was so bad that I could not really leave the party with her because she was throwing up almost every minute and there was no way to strap her in her car seat. As fast as it started it was over, it only lasted a few hours and then she seemed like she was fine. I figured it was just some crazy reaction to some new juice she had tried for the first time that night. She would never have any other symptoms when this would happen, no fever, no runny nose, nothing just puke everywhere. These events would happen here and there for the first three years of her life but were always blamed on something else. I didn't think much of those events because they did not happen that often and they didn't start really cycling on a regular basis until she hit three years old. Looking back at the whole picture now CVS makes so much more sense and explains it all.

She cycles almost exactly on the 12th or 13th of every month. Her cycle only lasts for six to eight hours, and it always happens a few hours after she falls asleep, but by morning she is fine. She's tired, but it's over. She has no known triggers, but we just started a journal a few months ago, so we are hopeful that that will help identify some of them. We are lucky her episodes aren't as severe as other children's episodes can be. At first we were told that it was not CVS due to it only lasting a few hours. I would love other parents that are searching for answers like I was to know that just because the vomiting may not be as severe as some, it definitely can still be CVS. We started bringing her to a chiropractor which seems to have cut her episodes way down in frequency and in severity. And that we homeschool her so she doesn't have to deal with coming in contact with so many germs. With homeschooling her, it allows us to rearrange our schedule so much easier when an episode does hit and it eliminates so much stress on her. We are hopeful that even though Irelynn has CVS that she will go on to live a pretty normal life.

Lizzie's Path: Help from a Cardiologist
Jenni Surface

A month before Lizzie turned three she became extremely ill and vomited non-stop for several hours. She was so sick that she threw up as much as ten times an hour. After about three hours she developed an extremely high temperature that went up to 105. She was hospitalized for what they thought was a virus. Little did we know, this was only the first episode of many we would see in the coming months.

The next episodes came every six to eight weeks and we were continually told it was a virus each time. As we grew frustrated from going in and out of the hospital and the doctors writing it off as a virus, we knew we needed to change something. I went to see my wonderful cardiologist for a checkup and he noticed my heart rate was up. He asked me what was wrong and I told him our story about Lizzie. He promptly got on the phone and found us the best pediatrician he could within the Duke system. We switched Lizzie to his care.

From there everything moved quickly. We had several tests run. We were directed to different specialist. Lizzie now had appointments to see a neurologist, a GI doctor, a psychologist, a geneticist, and a new pediatrician. She ended up back in the hospital again for five days after seeing all of them the first time. Her team worked so well together and it is then that we first started hearing the words *abdominal migraine*. New to us, and while it fit somewhat, it didn't fit everything that was going on with her. It would take another four months and several tests before they would diagnose her with Cyclic Vomiting Syndrome.

After reading about CVS, I finally felt we were headed in the right direction. I still was frustrated, but I felt closer to knowing how to help my daughter not suffer so much. We started a treatment plan, and at first it didn't seem to do anything. In fact, her episodes increased to once every two weeks. We finally started her on CoQ10 and L-carnitine along with the highest dose of cyproheptadine she could take. We have now seen a decrease in episodes.

She has episodes every four weeks now, and they do not end up in the hospital. We are able to manage them at home with Zofran. She still feels crappy during that time and has even shown differences in her behavior and energy levels. We are still a work in progress in this area and we are learning to adapt to accommodate her needs. Our family is always on edge because we never know when an ugly episode may come again and how she may handle it. I hope one day we will be able to help her continue to find answers and no longer have to remain on pins and needles.

Taylor's Path: Keeping a Journal
Rhonda Feasel

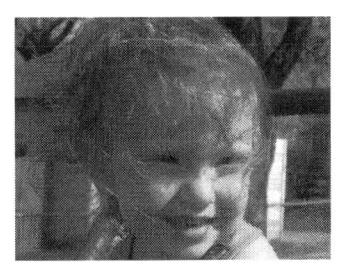

When I first found out that my daughter Jody and son-in-law Caleb were going to have a baby it was the most wonderful moment ever. My first grandbaby was on its way. I was so full of excitement and could not wait for the day I got to see and hold and love this little angel. She came a month earlier than expected. She was beautiful with her red hair and her big blue eyes. Just a Godsend to all of us! Taylor Renee was born in April of 2008 and her trials and tribulations started the day she was born. They had to keep her in the hospital a few more days than expected due to her sugar levels being low. But a few days later she was able to go home. And we were so happy that she was okay and healthy.

Then when she was three months old at one of her checkups they found a heart murmur and was sent to Children's Hospital in Columbus, Ohio for some testing on her heart. We were so scared and nervous waiting on the results from her heart test, but received a phone call a few days later saying that she was okay. She did have a murmur, but only a slight one. What a sigh of relief we had knowing that our little angel would be okay and could live a healthy, happy life. And she did, until she was about a year old.

She began having these episodes of vomiting, and not just vomiting like from a tummy bug or something, but vomiting every 20 minutes or so for days. And we knew something terrible was wrong with her. But we did not know what. I can remember the look in my daughter's eyes of worry and concern and exhaustion at what our little angel was going through, being put through all these tests and hooked up to all these machines. They did MRIs, CAT scans, heart testing, EEGs, blood work ups, Barium testing, endoscopies and colonoscopies and DNA testing.

Out of all these tests they did we came to find out she had a cyst on her pineal gland in her brain, she had a heart murmur and DNA showed that she was a carrier of ALFA ONE ANTITRYPCIN DISORDER, but none of these were the reason why she was vomiting so much. We were so scared for her, not knowing the seriousness of any of these findings. We were overwhelmed, and I know she was scared also, not knowing why we were doing this to her.

We cried so much after getting no answers from all the tests that they were doing, but we did not give up hope that they would find out what was wrong with Taylor, and neither did the doctors. They worked so hard to find an answer and finally one day we got our answer...not what we wanted, but we got an answer. They told us that Taylor had CVS—Cyclic Vomiting Syndrome.

We had never heard of this before and immediately started to educate ourselves on this disease. The first three years of her suffering from this kept us in and out of the hospital at least a week every month or every other two months. We watched as she suffered from these episodes and what she went through during them. For days on end she would just be laying there, lethargic and nonresponsive.

We worried so much. All the meds and teams of doctors that came in and out of her room and explaining to us what she was going through was overwhelming and hard to take in. As we got more educated on this and everything else that was going on we decided there were things we needed to do to be prepared for an episode. So we would have bags packed with extra clothing, tooth brushes and hairbrushes, deodorant, just stuff we would need to have to be gone for a while. We keep a journal just on her CVS:

- when it starts, how many times she vomits in a day and the times of the vomiting,
- what she ate or drank or how long it has been since she ate or drank
- how often she goes to the bathroom or NOT gone
- what meds we have given her and what time they were given and if she held them down
- trips to the hospital and what happened there.

When she started school we made a book for her to explain to the teacher, nurse, principal and bus driver what CVS is and how to help her if an episode occurs. We keep puke buckets in every vehicle she may ride in and one by her bed also. This is no way for a child to live. Taylor was a year old when diagnosed with CVS and she is six now. It has NOT gotten any easier for her or for us, but we do what we can to make her comfortable during an episode and let her know we are here for her.

CVS is not just a tummy bug that makes you vomit. It is an invisible disease, a monster that makes you throw up every 10 to 20 minutes for days. It leaves you in a lethargic state where you can't move, speak, or open your eyes. You just want to sleep so the pain in your stomach will stop and you want to be in a quiet, dark place. You dehydrate from all the vomiting and when you have thrown up everything in your stomach you start throwing up bile. You can't take anything by mouth for it will cause you to vomit again; you usually end up in the hospital anywhere from a few hours to a few days with IV fluids running through you to hydrate you and to feed you your meds. This disease is so horrible, so we need to raise awareness of CVS. We need a better understanding and we need research. We need you to help raise awareness of this invisible monster.

Leonie's Path: Dancing
Anne Van Vliet

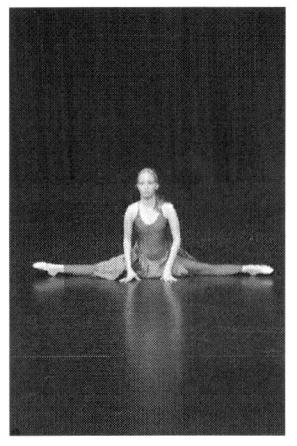

Leonie was born in September of 1998 in Australia. She was a full term baby but was very small and weighed only less than 5 lbs. Leonie has remained very small being just under five feet tall and weighing 88 pounds at age 16. Leonie would often vomit as a baby and by the time she was two she had several episodes of vomiting that lasted for more than a day and she started to be admitted to hospital for treatment for the vomiting and rehydration. It took only a few admissions before one of the pediatricians told us that he thought Leonie suffered from Cyclic Vomiting Syndrome.

They started her on preventative medicine and performed many tests. Over the next eight years Leonie would have been admitted to hospital about five times a year and have many more episodes that we dealt with at home. Leonie's cycles became less frequent as she got older and from about the age of 13 we could manage most episodes at home with medication with only the occasional need to be admitted to hospital.

As Leonie has reached puberty things have changed. She has started getting migraine headaches. Up until this point she would hardly ever get a headache but suddenly she could not get out of bed for days because of the pain and associated with them and they were making her feel nauseous. At the present time we are trying different migraine medicines to find what will work for her. So far the preventer that stops the headaches leaves her so fatigued that she can't think clearly or concentrate on her school work. The fatigue also triggers the nausea so she is back to being too sick to get out of bed most mornings. We are still in the trial stage so hopefully we can find the right dose to give her a balance and to get her to school more regularly.

Leonie's body does not seem to tell her that she is thirsty and she has never consumed enough fluids. We are always having to remind her about eating and drinking. At one stage Leonie was burning up more calories than she was consuming. Her appetite was not the best with always feeling nauseous as well as losing everything every time she vomited. She would also burn up a lot of energy with her ballet. We found out that this was causing ketones to build up in her body. The ketones building up would make Leonie feel nauseous so she wouldn't eat and drink meaning her body was burning any stored fat and causing more ketones to build up. After she was hospitalized one time and still had ketones present even after she had been on the drip the doctors suggested that Leonie should do what it takes to increase her calorie intake. She was told to have a chocolate bar and a sugary drink before a ballet class so that her body would have something to burn. We make sure she eats and drinks lots to keep her body hydrated and to have energy to burn and this has helped a bit. Fluids are a big key to keeping her well but she still has all of the other triggers such as excitement, stress, fatigue, viruses and other illnesses.

Leonie started doing ballet classes at the aged of five. These were very good for helping to build up her muscle strength and stamina. She has studied the Royal Academy of Dance Syllabus and this year she passed her Grade 8 exam with a distinction. This is an amazing feat for someone who could not get out of bed for the week before the exam. Leonie is lucky enough to have a very caring dance teacher who understood that Leonie was unwell and she would let her just watch the class if she was not well enough to dance. She would also give her catch up classes at her own house to help get her ready for an exam or competition. Leonie's teacher would never leave her out of a part in the concert or a competition troupe for fear of her not being well enough to turn up. She did miss one concert as she was in hospital and it really devastated her. A few times Leonie has taken the stage after coming out of hospital the day before but she was either in and episode and really sick or it had switched off and she was dancing again. One time she was vomiting on the way to a ballet exam, danced the exam and was admitted to hospital the next day but she was not going to let it stop her from passing her exam.

Leonie often wakes feeling nauseous and with the help of medication she often slowly improves as the day goes on. Even though she has not been well enough to go to school on these days, if it is a dance night we will still let her go and watch her ballet class or join in if she feels well enough. We think it is important not to let CVS spoil any more than it has to and try to let Leonie do everything other kids do. It is important for her mental wellbeing not to let her miss any more than she needs to. As a family we go on camping holidays with our family and friends. We camp up in the mountains on a farm by a river and go swimming and quad bike riding. We sit around the camp fire and play cards and board games. Leonie can do as much or as little as she likes. She can lay in her bed and rest or she can join in the fun. We are only a couple of hours away from the hospital if it is needed.

Leonie is not going to let CVS win. It wins some of the battles but Leonie is winning the war. With the support of family and friends, schools, teachers and tutors, doctors and nurses and all of the people involved her life Leonie is making the best of the good days and is being looked after on the bad ones.

Isaac's Path: Sensory Integration and CVS
Pamela Souter

Isaac was born sick. He was a two pound preemie. There were so very many issues with him in the first year of his life that it took a while to finally see that there was a pattern to everything. When he was about two years old, I decided to start documenting his episodes. It wasn't until a year after that that we were actually given his diagnosis of CVS. Just recently, I was reading though my old posts from my blog when he was in NICU.

The following is from my care page when he was fewer than two months old: "When I arrived at the hospital today, Isaac was lying in a pool of his own vomit and did not even seem to notice he had thrown up. He was non-responsive to the touch and seemed 'really out of it.' Along with many other issues, Isaac also has Sensory Processing Disorder. This makes him even more sensitive to sounds and vibrations. For a child with sensory issues who does not have CVS, the oversensitivity can be avoided by walking away from the stimulus. However, once Isaac has been overstimulated, it frequently sends him into an episode of CVS, which always ends up with him in the ER within five hours."

Every CVS person has a different cycle. I feel so blessed that his cycle is always over the worst part within 24 hours, and he's completely back to normal within 2 days. However, his cycle is so very violent and incapacitating. He not only cannot stop throwing up every few minutes, he cannot even lift his own head or speak. He fits the "conscious coma" profile perfectly. It is now at the point that he is experiencing so much anxiety about getting sick that he avoids many things that typical children do for fun, like swinging, listening to music, running around, and even swimming. I find, too, that he is at higher risk for getting sick when he is tired.

One of the most difficult aspects of being his mother is attempting to explain this disease to others. Nearly everyone I meet is unaware of the existence of this disease. It is hard to find a good balance of what to allow my child to experience, and when to draw the line and tell him he has to go to bed, or get out of the water, or calm down, without looking like I'm sheltering my child from having fun or living life to its fullest.

Trinity's Path: A Long Awaited Gift with Surprises
Tiffany Sharpe from Trinities Troops

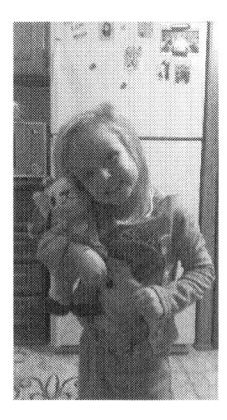

Well I should probably start from the very beginning. I got married at the age of 19 to the love of my life. I wanted to have children right away, but he wanted to wait. So we waited what seemed like forever! Then we decided to have a baby, as if it were only that easy. Sadly this pregnancy would end early at twelve weeks. It was the hardest thing I have ever had to go through. I was a mother with no child. So there we were back to square one, only now I am grieving. So we kept trying. It took us fifteen months.

I went to the doctor to see if she could put me on some fertility medicine and she made me take a pregnancy test. The wait seemed like a lifetime. The nurse came out to the waiting room and called me back. She showed me the test and I couldn't believe my eyes: I was pregnant! This time I had a beautiful baby girl named Trinity. Weighing in at six pounds eleven ounces and perfect. Although I had some complications and had to have an emergency C-section and she had to have an IV in her head the entire three days, I got to bring her home!

Things were going great until she was about six months old. She would projectile vomit a lot. Every time we would get her to the doctor the puking would be over. When she was about ten months old she was hospitalized for an ear infection and dehydration. After that she kept having these episode of vomiting. It started out about every three months, then they got closer and closer until they were two weeks apart and every time I made it to the doctor, she was done. We had a few ER visits for fluids and they became more and more frequent.

The pediatrician finally set us up with a GI doctor at All Children's Hospital. All I wanted was answers. With my first visit to the GI he said, "It sounds like acid reflux, but it could be cyclic vomiting syndrome." I left thinking it was acid reflux. He gave her prevacid. It seemed to help at first but the episodes kept happening, just a little farther apart. I even took her to her third birthday party with a puke bucket. I kept seeing him for about two years. He did an endoscopy and found gastritis and then did an MRI which came back clear.

He prescribed her nexium for the gastritis. He told me that it should heal up in about twelve weeks and if she has an episode after that then she has Cyclic Vomiting Syndrome. So here I was with those three words I knew nothing about. I went home and started my research. I couldn't believe how similar our situation was and how she fit all of the criteria. By this time she was four years old. Her GI wanted to refer me to Dr. Bi Li in Wisconsin. We live in Florida! So I contacted the Cyclic Vomiting Syndrome Association (cvsaonline.org) and they sent me a list of doctors in my area.

The closest doctor was four hours away in Jacksonville but it was better than Wisconsin. He is a geneticist and the appointment went great! He assured me I was making good choices in what we were doing for her episodes. He put her on LCarnitine and Zofran daily. So here we are, four years into our journey with CVS, and finally can put a name to it. She is now five years old and episode free for the past two months. Her episodes are mild compared to some, they last anywhere from four to twelve hours, during which she vomits every five to ten minutes. After six hours I know to take her to the ER for IV fluids. It is just getting to know your child when they are in an episode. We take this journey one day at a time until someday we find a cure.

Shun's Path: Will I Live to Be an Adult?
Shun Emoto

My name is Shun Emoto. I'm a 23-year-old graduate student of Japan. Since elementary school I've had cyclic vomiting syndrome. Once a week, I'll have an episode lasting 16 to 24 hours. These come with severe abdominal pain and five or six vomiting attacks per hour. The cycle starts with several hours of stomach pain, the vomiting and pain peaking at about the tenth hour. I can live normally when not in one of these cycles, but during an attack I have to keep hydrated and sleep as much as I can.

The diagnosis didn't come easy. My symptoms, including seizures, didn't fit with those typically associated with the flu. A urine test showed no abnormalities, so my doctor next examined my blood and then my brain waves. Perhaps my condition only needed therapy to overcome? I couldn't explain to my friends or my teachers why I was absent from school and in the hospital. I felt despondent. My anxiety increased. All I knew was that some unknown disease was horribly attacking me once a week.

When I was nine, my mother started taking notes on the times of my attacks and seizures. She suspected that the pain and vomiting had a pattern. She was right. We showed the notes to the doctor and he agreed. At this time, the hospital I went to began treating a girl with similar symptoms, and I opted to be admitted for testing as well. The hospital concluded that I had CVS.

With this diagnosis, we had a name attached to my symptoms and we were reassured that I wasn't deathly ill. We felt hope. I wouldn't die before becoming an adult. However, we still didn't have a lot of information and there was still no effective treatment. I still worried because I didn't know exactly when an attack would occur or if it would mean missing school trips and fun excursions. I felt guilty for missing tests at school and the impact the condition had on my family. They had to pick me up from school whenever I had an attack. Junior high was worse because the workload increased and I had to cram for tests and catch up on a lot of school work after being out. Studying ceased to be fun.

Worse yet was high school, a time when I had to be thinking about college entrance exams and my future. The hospital had told us that my disease would be cured by the time of puberty. When no changes came I grew very anxious. I avoided thinking about college, my career, and the possibility of marriage, fearful that my condition would prevent me from doing these things. Japan's social security system could help with costs, but it doesn't stop me from worrying that I wouldn't grow up properly. I had an attack three days before the college entrance exam, but things turned around when I moved to Tokyo. The symptoms went away. I don't know why.

I suffered from CVS for 12 years. It was often painful and always annoying. The information we had was very poor. I had no specialist to go and see. No one near me knew what I was going through. I couldn't share my pain with anyone who really understood. I knew of no associations I could join or meetings I could attend. I therefore started meetings myself and now do consultations with people based on my own experiences and also the information I've gained from CVSA in America. I hope to grow this network for people in Japan living with CVS.

Devon's Path: A Irish Tale
Amanda Doyle

It was back in 2009, when Devon was nine months old, that his symptoms first started. Though his condition seemed to present itself at first as a really strong stomach bug, it soon became very apparent that this was more than your average childhood stomach bug.

Devon awoke in his crib in the early hours of the morning crying uncontrollably. When I went to him and lifted him out of his crib he was extremely pale and projectile vomited everywhere. I called my husband to grab some towels and clean clothes for him, saying that it looked like he might have a tummy bug. I had seen a few tummy bugs in children due to already having an older son and two younger brothers. The whole time I held Devon he tried to wriggle out of my arms, so I set him down on the floor to clean his crib. He then, at nine months old, lay in the fetal position and curled himself up, which made me think he may have some abdominal pain. We brought him to our out-of-hours doctor as the vomiting continued without relent, and I was worried that it could be his appendix causing the tummy pain.

The doctor examined him and straight away, confirmed it was not appendicitis, and diagnosed a tummy bug. He advised us to hold off giving him food and to just keep pushing fluids. We headed home, where the vomiting continued relentlessly for 48 hours, but we just assumed that it was a tummy bug that just needed to work its way out of his system. On the third day, although tired and quiet, Devon awoke and the vomiting had stopped. Color had returned to his face and his energy levels were working themselves back up to his lively, boisterous self. It was the worst case of vomiting I had seen in a tummy bug ever and I was dreading myself or my husband or our eldest son getting this. Because that's what happens, isn't it? Stomach bugs are contagious, right?

It never happened, though. No one else in our house got this so called tummy bug.

A few weeks later Devon awoke vomiting exactly the same way again, for the same length of days, but this time he started to vomit up bile and we ended up in A&E (Accident and Emergency, the Irish term for what in the U.S. is called the ER, the Emergency Room). He was deathly pale, lethargic, with dark circles under his eyes, vomiting at a max nine times an hour, curled up with an obvious pain in his tummy and drooling excessively.

Blood tests revealed he was dehydrated so much they struggled to find a vein even though we had been administering plenty of fluids including rehydration solutions we bought from the pharmacy.

The IV solution they gave him for dehydration gave him a long enough break in the vomiting to go asleep. He slept for hours and when he awoke the vomiting had stopped exactly 48 hours after it began (same as last time). The hospital doctor again said it was a tummy bug or some sort of virus. I told my husband I wasn't happy with them fobbing us off with this diagnosis, but he asked me why I would question a doctor's medical training. Again no one in our home contracted this stomach bug.

When it happened again another few weeks later I was astounded. How can my little boy keep getting these stomach bugs? Is his immune system that bad? Why was no one else in our house getting it too? Could it be gluten intolerance (his daddy's mother is a celiac)?

All these questions went through my mind. It was when I took out a calendar and marked off the dates he had his first vomiting episode, the second, and now this one, that I noticed that these episodes were exactly four weeks apart all the time. Not every time would take us to A&E, but the vomiting continued for the same amount of time and all symptoms would be always the same. I decided then to keep a diary of his episodes if they continued to happen and I began some research in the internet, looking for possible causes for episodes of relentless vomiting that was constantly diagnosed as a stomach bug but seemed way worse than that.

Towards the end of 2010 the frequency of his episodes had changed to every few months, but the duration started to increase to 72 hours or more. Every time, even though his medical history showed repeated episodes of vomiting, it was always the same diagnosis: a stomach bug.

A Dublin hospital even went as far as having him referred to a psychologist, suggesting he was doing this to himself and it was some sort of behavioral thing. This is when I came across a forum on the internet about a condition that caused episodes of unexplained, severe, relentless nausea and vomiting. I read thousands of stories from other people that had children just like Devon. I even read stories of adults that suffered with the same symptoms as Devon. Slowly the jigsaw pieces to the puzzle of why my son kept getting sick started to fit together. This condition was called Cyclical Vomiting Syndrome (CVS).

During my research, I came across two charities for CVS: CVSA in the UK and CVSA in the USA. During this time Devon's episodes continued but were now happening more sporadically. I was even beginning to notice warning signs of an episode about to happen. My child, who is always on the go and a typical noisy toddler, would go suddenly as quiet as a mouse, the colour would drain from his face and he would yawn constantly. Within 30 minutes of these warning signs happening he would begin the profusely relentless vomiting which would switch to dry retching once his stomach was empty. He would become so weak and lethargic. He was two now so he could show me where is tummy hurt. He never objected to having to go to hospital and without so much as a fuss let the nurses take bloods and put in IV lines. You can imagine how sick a child must feel to not even kick up a fuss to have injections!

By the time of my last visit to the hospital before Devon's official diagnosis I was aware of CVS but did not have the faith in the hospital medical professionals to bring this to their attention without back up from my GP. When I had gathered all my research I presented it to our family doctor and told her my concerns and that I felt the constant diagnosis of a stomach bug was wrong, my motherly instincts were screaming at me to look into this more and finally I came across CVS.

She read the paperwork I had brought with me and admitted that in all her years as a doctor and during all her time in medical school she had never heard of CVS. She agreed it could be a possibility that Devon could have this and agreed to refer me to a Gastroenterology team in Crumlins children's hospital. Whilst we awaited our appointment,

Devon was sent for all sorts of tests to rule out other possible causes of episodes of vomiting. He was tested for celiac disease, gutmalrotation, and he had upper GI tests performed, full blood workups, ultrasounds and x-rays. All tests came back negative for other conditions that could be found with diagnostic testing.

In early 2012, armed with Devon's episode diary, information on CVS, and information on our family medical history, it was finally time to see a gastroenterologist. We met with the doctor in Crumlin who did a full physical exam on Devon, reviewed Devon's medical history and reports from all tests performed, and spoke to me about my family medical history to the best of my knowledge. After an hour or so with this amazing doctor my son was diagnosed with CVS. He was given a prescription for Zofran as an abortive measure as by the time the appointment came around the doctor and I had agreed that Devon no longer suffered frequently enough to require a preventive medication. Even though the confirmed news of my son having this condition was awful I felt a huge weight lifted off my shoulder. I was not mad for thinking the doctors were wrong with their diagnosis of stomach bugs and my son was not doing this to himself due to behavior problems.

After the diagnosis I got in touch with the point of contact in Ireland as per the CVSA UK website. I spoke to her various times, and during our last correspondence, when I told her I would love to raise more awareness in Ireland about CVS, she informed me that she was retiring and asked would I be interested in taking her place as the CVS point of contact for Ireland. As my son was never an extreme case and his episodes have decreased a lot I jumped on this opportunity to take over this position and try raise the much needed awareness of CVS. I don't want other parents to go through years and years waiting on a diagnosis and I don't want sufferers to feel alone with this. This is a battle that is better fought together, so with this motivation I founded CVS Ireland in January 2014 and created an Irish support group on Facebook.

Joe's Path: Traveler's Blessing
Joe Meiners

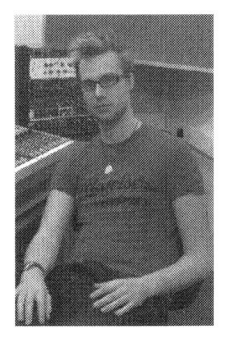

I remember my first bout of CVS when I was about seven years old. It lasted eight days. My mum had to do everything for me; I couldn't walk or sit up. I could barely talk. None of us had any idea that this was going to be my life for several years to come. Finally my GP agreed that it was time for him to see me and immediately I was hospitalized for dehydration.

My sickness continued in hospital whilst they tried to get the drug balance right with tablets that you swallowed, tablets that dissolved inside your lip, suppositories, etc., and I think I had a drip to rehydrate me, although it's all a bit of a blur now. Finally, the best thing that worked was Ondansetron, intravenously in the back of my hand. My sickness stopped within an hour or so and I felt back to normal with no side effects at all—except for being hungry! Over the next couple of years, this started to happen more and more. It's difficult to explain to someone who hasn't suffered with this, but the sickness and feelings of not being able to walk or talk well were obvious to me. It wasn't like a sick bug or something I'd eaten—I knew straight away and off we'd go to the doctor and then into hospital.

It was very frustrating because I've always been tall, and at age nine my mum couldn't carry me into the doctor's surgery any more. One day she got me to the car park and no further—the receptionists were beckoning her to carry me in but she just couldn't manage. Fortunately my GP happened to look out the window and realized what was happening so he came down, got on the floor next to me, and diagnosed me—as usual, straight into hospital. After this episode, my mum kicked up a fuss and said we went to hospital EVERY time so surely something could be done. Eventually the hospital agreed and gave us 'Open Access' to the children's ward. We only had to ring them direct and say we were on our way and they'd be ready for me.

Although this was so much better, when you're feeling really rough it could be frustrating too. Each time I went in they had to weigh me (I usually lost about 10 lbs in 24 hours even though there isn't much of me to start with), measure my height, etc., and then I'd have to wait for the doctor to be called as it was usually during the night I'd start being ill. He could take a couple of hours to arrive and then they'd talk through my medical history. It was so annoying because we'd say over and over that I needed Ondansetron in the back of my hand and I would go without magic cream. A few times I fell lucky and it would be the same registrar as my previous visit and I'd be home within two hours. One time it happened during the night between Christmas Day and Boxing Day—the rest of my family didn't even know I'd gone and wondered why we were tired!

One of the quickest treatments I had was in Turkey—no messing about. It was a family holiday with extended family which had been bequeathed to us. We got the best flight times we could for me, but it triggered another episode within an hour of arriving. Fortunately there was a good medical centre on site. My mum explained that I had a headache in my tummy and it wasn't the sun, and gave them our room number. Within 20 minutes a paramedic arrived, put up a drip (on the picture hook above the bed after removing the picture) with Ondansetron my arm went really cold where it pushed through so fast, but I was in the pool 50 minutes later with my family!

My 'episodes', as they were called, were far worse in the winter, and we linked them to tiredness. If I had disturbed sleep from a cold, I would almost be able to guarantee a bout of CVS and a few trips to the children's ward. At least it gave me a chance to help myself a bit where I could. I saw the pediatrician at my local hospital who diagnosed various drugs for me over the next few years but none of them worked (unless I wanted to be asleep at school – which did happen on a few occasions). I preferred to be normal and deal with the episodes than be a zombie. Eventually I was told that I had to just 'manage it myself', there was nothing more that could be done by the NHS. By this time, school was getting difficult. I frequently vomited on my way to school, during lessons, during exams—this was on top of the episodes so everyday life was getting to be a challenge.

At this time, my step-mum found that she could add me on her private health care scheme and my GP (understanding how bad it was) said she would refer me to whomever I wanted. I am very fortunate to have seen a doctor who was really caring and gave me some hope. I had lots of tests involving biopsies, standing on one leg with my eyes shut in a blacked out room with an infrared camera on my eyes watching my movement, etc. Eventually they realized that my body was dizzy all the time. On the outside I was still but inside it was like I lived on a roller coaster, which is why I was sick frequently. I was referred to a vestibular physiotherapist in London, and after only a single session and a week of strange exercises, I was able to notice an improvement.

I had to make myself dizzy for my body to learn to correct itself so I did things like bending over with my hands on the floor and bottom in the air and shaking my head from side to side quite vigorously. It was very frustrating—had the tests been carried out when I was seven, I could have been spared lots of illness, hospital visits, embarrassment, etc. for seven years. Had I known about these tests earlier, I would have given them a try.

I am now about 95% improved and take no regular drugs. I still have days when I feel queasy, but I can manage it. I sat my GCSEs, A levels and am now at university. Don't give up hope!

When It's CVS Plus....

Sometimes Cyclic Vomiting Syndrome is the only medical condition our kids suffer from. However, there are kids who are known to have "CVS plus." These kids suffer from seizure disorders, autism or autism-like symptoms, mitochondrial disease and many other conditions which can make treatment and management more difficult. Some have feeding tubes, developmental delays, or a host of other symptoms.

Actually, my family falls into this category with Andrew's diagnosis of CVS, autism spectrum and anxiety. Finding families who also struggled with other conditions that seem at times to feed the cyclic vomiting was a breath of fresh air. These families can relate to how there is no one simple answer or treatment and that we need more than just medicine. We often encounter others who fail to grasp the complexity that CVS is in our lives. There are so many pieces to the puzzle to sort out. It's more of a balancing act for us than it is for others with just CVS. It can come with hidden advantages, such as feeding tubes that can get meds into the body without a fight.

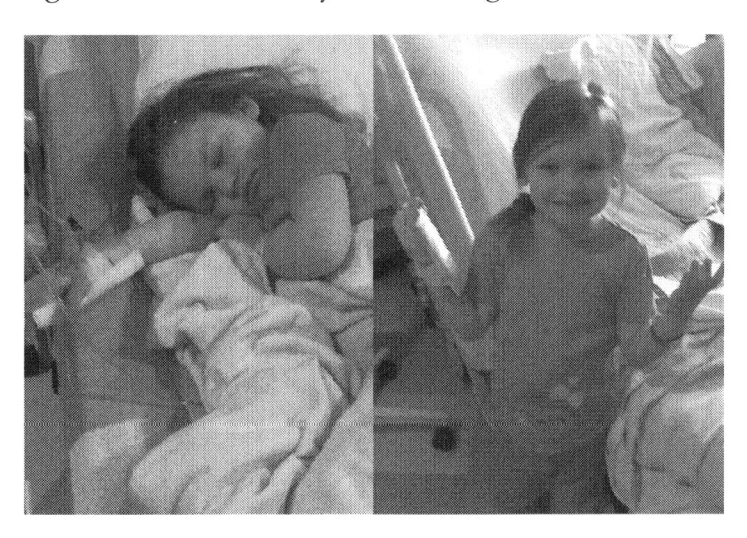

Hope's Path: CVS and Feeding Tubes
Melissa Knight

I shared my daughter's story of CVS with www.feedingmatters.org in the hope of educating more people about the challenges that we as CVS parents face.

My daughter experiences episodes of nausea, vomiting, severe retching, exhaustion, paleness, mild body aches, and extreme abdominal pain. Her known trigger is the common cold or virus, but sometimes a simple car ride can also be a trigger. She started with CVS at four months old with her very first cold. It was difficult to get a diagnosis for the vomiting since she recently had an NG tube put in place and had severe reflux. I initially thought the retching and gagging was from the NG tube along with the drainage in her throat from the cold.

Soon I realized that every head cold led to vomiting. I decided to closely document these episodes to find the diagnosis. I began tracking when colds began, when vomiting started, and what occurred immediately before and after episodes. After one and a half years of carefully documenting on calendars, I transferred all of the information to a journal and took it into the doctor to show him the pattern. It was then that she was diagnosed with CVS and treatment began. I was not happy to learn this diagnosis and it is not a definite answer because many other syndromes mimic CVS. It is a diagnosis of elimination. I have a strong understanding of this vicious cycle and this knowledge empowers me.

As my daughter grew older, the episodes worsened and hospitalization was needed with each cold. Prior to an episode starting, my daughter becomes extremely pale. She would become physically exhausted to the point that she cannot even sit up straight. Sometimes she would complain of a sore throat. I immediately give her medications to try to arrest the episode before it begins. As a mother I felt completely helpless. Then the stomach pain begins to set in and the screaming and moaning starts. She screams for me to make her stomach stop hurting and there is not one thing I can do but hold her and love her, so I place a cool washcloth on her forehead and hold her tight.

The vomiting starts right after the stomach pain begins. This continues consecutively until there is nothing left but air in her stomach. After her stomach is emptied, she begins retching. Besides the extreme pain, the retching is what bothers me the most. Her stomach continues to spasm, making the retching seem never ending. It is forceful and looks violent. Blood vessels normally pop out all around her eyes. As soon as the retching and pain turns into a twenty minute interval, we make our way to the hospital. I keep a pre-packed suitcase filled with medications and tube feeding supplies along with clothes and toys. It only took one time of being unprepared and trying to pack in the middle of the night to figure this out.

We start out in the emergency room where I have to be a strong advocate and push for an admission right away. The doctors try to make me tube feed her Pedialite just to see if she is going to vomit. I refuse to do that because all it does is start the violent cycle all over again. Now, we get admitted every time and the length of the hospital stay ranges from three to eight days. It varies depending on the abdominal pain, and when and how much Pedialite she can tolerate through her tube. Then we progress to watered down formula in her tube and so on.

When dealing with CVS, treatment plans change hourly. With that comes changing the doctor's orders. When the line of communication between myself and the doctor is left open, we get out of the hospital quicker. It is my job to advocate for my daughter when I find it necessary to, even if it means paging the doctor several times a day. Sometimes my instincts know to progress slower than what the doctor originally ordered and other times, I know I can speed up and increase the time and amount of tube feeds. Communication is necessary.

There is absolutely nothing in the world worse than seeing your child in pain and screaming for you to take the pain away. It is a heavy burden to carry. It is my job to comfort my children through their most difficult days and to show them strength on the outside. I save the breaking down until I am behind closed doors. Sometimes just being there, holding my child is all I can do. I have to remind myself that it does bring them comfort even though I feel helpless.

CVS makes dealing with the feeding disorder more difficult because every episode of CVS sets back the progress we made with eating. It is also difficult to maintain a healthy balance between allowing my daughter to live a well-rounded life outside of our house, and protecting her health and progress she is making with eating. So far, that balance has not been found, although, I am sure it will one day. Until then, I make our home as fun as I can and we take advantage of the summer months when viruses are not as severe.

Doctors are just beginning to learn of this syndrome and much more research is needed. Treatment plans need to be made if your child has CVS because there is no cure and medicines work differently on each person, and unfortunately, with each episode. Plans need to be changed as your child's episodes change. It is incredibly important to raise awareness so research can continue. There is a emerging connection between CVS and mitochondrial diseases and dysfunctions. Testing is expensive and often times inconclusive. This is why further research is needed to discover better treatment options or to find a cure. Since there is no known cure for CVS, my daughter's future remains in limbo regarding removing her feeding tube. Continuing with feeding therapy, and increasing her desire to eat, only strengthens my hope for her to eat quickly again after a CVS episode. I also hope, with more research, that one day, a cure will be found!

Thomas' Path: CVS and Autism
Amanda Marshall

It was at my 12 week scan I was told that my baby would be monitored for low birth weight issues. My doctor wasn't concerned so neither was I. My 20 week scan didn't go so smoothly and I was asked to come into the 'little room' for a chat. The sonographer explained that my baby only had a two vessel umbilical cord instead of the usual three. Together with the low PAPP-A we were expecting a very low birth weight. My doctor monitored us both closely throughout the rest of my pregnancy and five days before my due date the flow through the cord was compromised and I was induced. Sixteen hours later I gave birth to the most beautiful 'little' boy I had ever seen, Thomas. He's all limbs, the nurse told me, 53 cms long but only 2.5 kg. He was perfect.

I still remember the moment when my world seemed to stop, I was in the doctor's office staring at an X-Ray of my 12 month old son. I can't even remember blinking, but I do remember the tears flowing, wondering how could my baby walk with his spine in this mess. Thomas had a very rare form of Scoliosis—Congenital. His spine had not formed correctly in utero. Our orthopedic surgeon explained that Thomas had a complex scoliosis with three hemi-vertebrae in the thoracic region and one butterfly vertebrae in his neck. We were told that surgery to correct the curve was only a matter of time. Thomas will eventually need his spine to be fused and titanium rods inserted into his back to correct the curve. It's not ideal performing this type of surgery on children that are still growing so his surgeon is monitoring the curve at this stage. We are hoping to get through puberty before surgery needs to be performed.

Thomas is a genius. I can still hear others saying this to me: "Have you ever known a child to count like him?! He's unbelievable." From an early age Thomas *really liked* numbers. I mean there's like and there's LIKE and he was definitely the latter. He recited the numbers on the license plates of cars when we drove, he'd buy packets of numbers or books about numbers from the shops and would play with them for hours. He could count to 100 at age two. I never really noticed that he didn't seem to play with regular toys that much. He was my first so I had nothing to compare to. I never noticed that he conversed really well with adults but not so well with children. I mean most of our time was spent speaking with doctors and nurses so it was no wonder he related to them. It was after he'd started school that one of the teachers expressed her concern for his behaviour and mannerisms.

I was a little annoyed at first, wondering what they wanted from him. He was performing well at school, did it really matter that he liked numbers so much? It became obvious that something was different when he bought home some work that he'd completed at school, every page had numbers written all over the back. In no particular order just covered from one side to the other. I thought it a little odd but it wasn't until he had his first 'bad' meltdown that I realized we needed some help. We were in a cake shop looking for some icing colours when Thomas saw some number cookie cutters.

"I want them!" he shouted.

"No," I said. "We don't need them."

He threw himself on the floor, kicking, screaming and hitting out. It took all my strength to pick him up and drag him out of the store, totally embarrassed that everyone was looking at us. I could feel them staring, shocked and disgusted with his behaviour. He screamed the whole way home, kicking the back of the seat and in obvious distress. When we got home he finally calmed down and went off to play. I sat on the bathroom floor crying.

Thomas was diagnosed with High Functioning Autism just before his sixth birthday. It was like someone had opened my eyes. I finally saw all the struggles he had been having. His lack of eye contact, understanding questions that were asked of him and how to play with other kids.

We started early intervention straight after his diagnosis, Occupational Therapy and Speech Therapy. The changes in him since we started are amazing. His eye contact is much better, he can understand and recognize feelings, and he has made some good friends at school. He is still struggling with inferential comprehension but he is getting help at school and home. Having autism has made explaining CVS to him that bit harder. He has a real fear of needles and trying to explain why he needs another needle in a way that he understands has been virtually impossible.

Thomas had his first vomiting episode at around 15 months. He woke in the morning and was unusually quiet. He wouldn't eat his breakfast but was drinking water like he hadn't had any for days. The vomiting started really quickly. At first it was only a few vomits but it soon was clear he was really unwell and getting severely dehydrated. It was after he'd been vomiting continuously for over an hour that we piled him into the car and drove him straight to the Children's Hospital. He was given an IV and spent the next two days in hospital recovering. At this stage we had no idea that this was to become an all too familiar occurrence. Over the next few years Thomas was in and out of hospital regularly, always being diagnosed with Gastroenteritis. It got to the point that I'd hear someone had a tummy bug and I'd consider putting a Hazmat sign on our front door so no-one would come near us for fear Thomas would catch it.

It was on the eve of his third birthday party when he woke up with the usual dark circles and acetone smell on his breath that I knew something wasn't quite right. He wasn't keen on eating so I didn't push it. The vomiting didn't start for a few hours but when it did it was worse than any of the other vomiting episodes he'd had. This time he was vomiting brown stuff. I had no idea what it could have been but my fear was that it was feces. Thomas had struggled with constipation from very early on and I was worried he'd become so constipated that the only way he could pass a stool was to vomit it.

I packed the car and headed to the ER as I had done so many times before. I always took Thomas to the same hospital, and each time I'd worry that the doctors were going to think I had Munchausen's! I gave the ER doctor the towel he'd been vomiting the brown stuff on to be tested. The results showed that it was old blood. My poor little boy had nothing else left in his tummy so he was now vomiting blood. He was admitted for two days and put on an IV. It was hearing everyone at his party singing him happy birthday over the phone while we were stuck in hospital that lit a fire under me. I swore I'd find out why my little boy had had so many episodes of vomiting with no diarrhea.

After countless tests and one idiot doctor after another, we found an amazing Gastroenterologist, and Thomas was finally diagnosed with CVS. He was five. It was a relief to hear the words really, after so many hospital stays, IVs galore and ER doctors telling me it was ANOTHER gastro bug. I remember looking at him when he explained what CVS was and thinking how on earth could this child survive any more vomiting. There was nothing left of him. He was skin and bones, the acid build up in his mouth was causing him pain, and the dark circles under his eyes were like sinkholes.

But it's two years later and my boy is happy and healthy, weighing in at 32 kgs at his last check-up!!! He takes daily medication to prevent episodes and help him gain weight. He still suffers from them occasionally (mainly the headache with only a few vomits) but our life has changed for the better. We treat episodes with an Ondansetron (Zofran) wafer (which we have nicknamed 'The Miracle' wafer) and take it with us when we travel now too. Extreme tiredness sets Thomas off so we try to ensure he gets enough sleep every night and try not to plan too many things in one day. I'm not sure what the future holds but I'd like to think that one day Thomas will no longer require medication, but at this stage we are happy that he's been IV free for almost 12 months!

Derek's Path: Cyclic Vomiting Syndrome and Autism
Beth Hanson

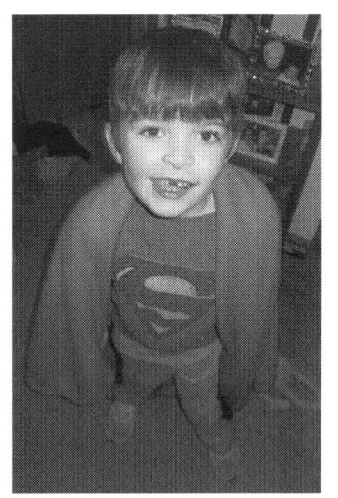

It is 3:05 a.m. Derek makes a coughing noise. I instantly wake up, and check him. He's still asleep. He coughs again. I ask if he's ok. I get no answer. I put my head back down on the pillow and try to sleep. 3:10 a.m. Derek gags. I sit up. I ask Derek if he's going to throw up. Too late. Vomit shoots out of his mouth. I pick him up and run for the bathroom. It's not far. I hold him over the toilet as he retches, uncontrollably. This will continue every 10-15 minutes for the next 4-5 hours. It happens almost every month. This is Cyclic Vomiting Syndrome. This is our life.

One of the biggest challenges for Derek (and for me) when he gets sick (not just with a CVS episode) is that Derek cannot tell me he is feeling ill. He can't tell me what hurts. He can't tell me when his head hurts or his stomach hurts or his ear hurts. I have to watch for signs. Sometimes he'll pull on his ear or go to bed early or just not eat anything when he is sick. But, unfortunately, sometimes he does these things when he's perfectly fine too, so I don't really have a good indication that my son is sick unless he has a fever or is vomiting.

When it comes to CVS, most people have some indication that an episode is coming on. Some people see an aura. Some become more sensitive to lights or noise. Most have stomach pain or headaches or both. I don't know if my son experiences any of that. I am assuming he does, but since he is autistic and has sensory processing disorder, I know that he's sensitive to lights and noise and crowds and tastes and smells all the time anyway. So is it even more extreme before a CVS episode? I don't know. Perhaps. ~~I wish I could ask him~~. No. Strike that. I wish he could answer.

I *do* know that when he is in the middle of an episode, and he gets vomit on himself, he can't stand it. He freaks out because the vomit is wet and gross. He doesn't like the way it feels to vomit either. He cries and asks me for help. It breaks my heart, because there is nothing I can do. He also is extra sensitive to the feeling of fabric on his skin and wants it off immediately. He prefers to be completely naked, and in between rounds of vomiting, he sleeps on the bathroom floor on piles of blankets and towels.

We have been lucky. Derek hasn't had to be hospitalized yet because of dehydration. I dread when he is more than you can possibly imagine. Derek can't stand IVs and will most likely yank it out of his arm. He also hates wearing hospital bracelets.

On the plus side, medication has helped Derek tremendously. At one point he was having episodes once a week. Now he has them maybe once a month; if we are lucky once every two months. I'm also hoping that as he gets older and more aware of his body, he'll be able to tell me when he's feeling sick, and he'll be able to take the appropriate "abort" medicines to avoid episodes altogether.

I cross my fingers that the episode is over. 7:45 a.m. Derek is asleep on the bathroom floor. His face is white as a sheet. I carry his limp body to the bed and cover him with a blanket. I kiss his clammy forehead. I wish I could sleep too, but I have about five loads of laundry to do. Vomit laundry. The bathroom is trashed. I also have to get Tyler to school. My day has just begun...

http://autismartproject.blogspot.com

Natalie's Path: Diagnosis of CVS Plus Mitochondrial Disease
Nicole Dion

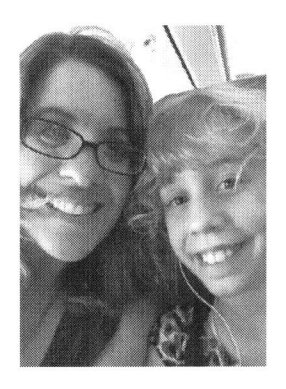

Mike and I received a call from Natalie's amazing new doctor in San Francisco. He was ready to share the preliminary results from the muscle biopsy she had just a couple weeks ago. I listened to all he had to say and then... *I cried.*

I cried because he told us that her preliminary test results confirmed a mitochondrial disease diagnosis, and our glimmer of hope that maybe we, and the various physicians who had given her that working diagnosis, were wrong.

I cried because he told us that it is not be something she will "grow out of" as we were first told a few years ago. Instead, her body will face a slow progression with the speed dependent on many things including her adherence to her treatment and protocol, as well as her avoidance of any major illnesses and hits to her immune system.

I cried because of the outstanding questions about her prognosis that remain, and will hopefully be better answered when we get the results of the more extensive testing on her muscle tissue that is being completed at two different hospitals. And...for those questions that will be unable to be answered because of the nature of the condition.

I cried because this is not the journey I would desire for her. But most of all...

I cried because I was glad that after eleven years of atypical medical issues with Natalie (with the last four years having been increasingly challenging for her), and test after test that was "inconclusive" but clearly not normal, we finally have a definitive diagnosis that we can stand on, and move forward with.

I cried because we don't have to worry about prideful, ignorant doctors trying to tell us that my daughter's issues are "in her head" or a result of anxiety of some other psychological root cause. I felt relief. We no longer have to debate with doctors, or live in as much fear that our daughter could be taken away such as happened with Justina Pelletier with a presumed mitochondrial disorder. We have been following her case since October with a clear realization that her story could be OUR story. My heart breaks for her family. Doctors disagreed about Justina's medical diagnosis of mitochondrial disease and instead felt her parents were to blame. Boston Children's Hospital then removed her from her parents care for over a year and removed all medical treatments. It took a media storm of appeals and petitions to get her eventually released back to her parents care.

I cried because I know there are so many other kids out there like Natalie who are misdiagnosed and/or not getting the proper treatment resulting in a horrible quality of life, or sometimes, even death. Mitochondrial disease and dysfunction are a rapidly growing. This is simply due to the lack of knowledge and awareness even within the medical community. This has to change.

I cried because I realized how much our previous neurologist endangered my daughter's health when, instead of figuring out how to proceed and consulting with someone else, he called me to tell me that he was "throwing his hands up," didn't know what else to do, and abandoned her care while she was still suffering and medically compromised, and in her 10th week of a migraine episode for which she had been hospitalized twice for with no relief this past October.

I cried because in losing her previous neurologist, we were led to Natalie's new neurologist, who has overwhelmed us with his kindness, tremendous knowledge, and such thorough support and care we almost don't even know how to receive it.

I cried because we were only able to see this neurologist and all of his fellow doctors who are supporting Natalie's care because we were forced to pick new insurance (and doctors) after Mike's work told us that they were dropping our current insurance plan, causing us to panic at the thought of losing the primary doctor and hospital that Natalie has had for her entire life.

I cried because our new doctors (and hospital) are knowledgeable and have done more for Natalie (and us) in the last four months than has been done in all of these years. They "get it," and we don't have to plead her case, educate them, or spur them on. They educate us and advocate on her behalf. They provide "active care," and meet our needs before we even ask. This brings me such comfort.

I cried because we got to experience God "moving us" when we were stuck in our comfort zone, unaware of the next steps to take. It was painful and hard, requiring us to take a deep breath and "step off the boat." We did it, and the results have been beyond our expectations. Our first step was moving her care to the hospital in San Francisco, forcing her (and us) to leave the familiar "home away from home" we had had at our hospital in Sacramento for the last eleven years. It is a place we were so very comfortable at, one full of nurses and Child Life staff who have provided great care and so much love to my sweet girl for all of these years. This move, coupled with changing insurances and all of Natalie's physicians (including her primary doctor) was the best thing that could have happened. The difference in Natalie's medical care and the coordination between doctors far surpasses what I even knew was possible. That is not to say our previous hospital and doctor(s) did not care or desire to help her; they simply did not have the knowledge required to properly handle her situation.

I cried for these and many other unwritten reasons after we talked with the doctor because there is so much wrapped up in all of this. So many mixed emotions, so much to carry and then surrender as we move through it. Even with the challenges, I feel so very blessed.

And I am crying now because my heart is full and thankful, for all that has gone on, and is to come, and for the many people who love and pray for my daughter. She inspires me, and brings me joy and laughter, even on the more challenging days. I do not know why this road was chosen for her, but I know she will continue to bring light and love as she travels it. We know not what the future holds, but we do know God will be with us on the journey.

Betsy's Path: Feeding Tubes, CVS and Teen Years
Connie Carrol

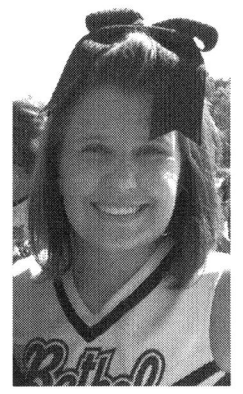

Betsy is currently 15 and was diagnosed with Cyclic Vomiting Syndrome when she was 14. She first became sick when she was 13 in November of 2012. When she had her first episode her dad and I just thought she had a really bad virus. It was a little different than a typical virus due to the fact we had never seen anyone vomit for so many hours at a time. With this episode came a severe sharp stabbing pain in her back that ended up moving around her side to her stomach. This episode occurred on a Thursday night and by the next Friday she was sick again.

This time I took her to her PCP because it seemed a little weird to me to have two viruses within a week of each other. I was just told that could happen and to make sure I keep her hydrated. Again, she had another episode in another week, so I took her back to the doctor and was told the same thing. On the fourth episode, after calling her doctor asking for some kind of help, we took her to the ER of our children's hospital. I was furious by the time I left. Not only did we have to wait six hours while she was vomiting, but the doctor who saw Betsy told me she was just constipated. I tried to explain that couldn't be the case, and even though I know my daughter better than anyone, she still would not listen to me.

Of course, another episode occurred four days later, so we went back to the ER. This time they told us Betsy had acid reflux, so we went home with her still sick and vomiting. The next day the ER contacted me, and said they thought they found a kidney stone and had us return. After making the trip back they said it wasn't and stuck with acid reflux. Finally on December 23, when Betsy had another episode, we saw a doctor in the ER who realized something was really wrong and was very concerned about Betsy's 20 pound loss. Betsy is only 5'2" and only weighed about 118 before getting sick so she didn't need to lose 20 pounds.

She was in the hospital for a week and had many different tests. The only one that showed anything was the test they did to check the functions of her gall bladder. The test was very painful and Betsy got sick during and after. It showed that her gall bladder was not functioning at all, but there was no known reason why. The surgeons decided to treat her instead of taking it out so we started meds and headed home. We were home two days until she was back in the hospital. This time they removed her gall bladder. We were so hoping it would take care of everything even though we weren't sure this was her problem.

After the surgery, Betsy did pretty well for about two weeks, and then it all started again. This time her GI doctor decided to put an NJ tube in due to all the weight loss and to give her stomach a rest. Her doctor strongly felt like this had something to do with narrowing of her ducts, so they sent her to The Children's Hospital in Philadelphia to their GI clinic. Again, Betsy had many, many tests done. Her doctor there diagnosed her with Autonomic Intestinal Neuropathy and began treating her with Amitriptyline. Still with the feeding tube we went home with as many or more questions than before. The Amitriptyline seemed to help so the tube came out in April. She had a great summer with some pain, but no vomiting. We thought it might be over.

However, in September, Betsy had another episode and was hospitalized. During this visit her doctor ordered a blood test to be done the next time she went into the ER with an episode. While hospitalized again in October and after the results from the blood work she was finally diagnosed with CVS. She stayed on the same meds but they were increased, and she had a great couple of months. When January came she was in the hospital every four to five days. After five hospital stays and lots of frustration we went back to CHOP in February. While we were there she had another extremely bad episode and was hospitalized for a week. During this time her doctor changed her meds from Amitriptiline to Phenobarbitol. We went home with the feeding tube which she kept until the beginning of May.

While Betsy has the tube she seems to do very well. It's July 4, 2014 now, and until this past week she had not had a full blown episode since March. While in the hospital we discussed putting in a port. She is 15 and hates having a tube in her nose. Not very stylish to a teenage girl. She is also on her school's cheer squad so she would be able to still cheer and have it at the same time.

Unfortunately we have not been able to get Betsy's pain under control and that always comes before the vomiting. It's very frustrating and heartbreaking to see my 15 year old hurt all of the time. She was a healthy child who all of a sudden went from having sleep overs and hanging out with friends to having pain, vomiting, feeding tubes and being in and out of the hospital constantly.

We are currently trying a new medicine at home when her pain starts in addition to the Tramadol, Ativan, and Zofran. It's a Synera pain patch she puts directly on her back where the pain is. She also has Sumatriptan 20mg which is a nose spray for pain. She doesn't take it very often due to the taste - it seems to make her more nauseated.

Betsy also takes enzymes that have been known to help with CVS. CO Q-10 - 100mg /3 x's day, L-Carnitine - 1,000mg/3 x's day, along with B-6 and Magnesium 1 x day. All of these are taken in addition to her Phenobarbital, Prilosec, and Zantac, and the meds she takes when she has pain.

The number one thing I have learned throughout this process is that I am the one that has to make sure my child gets what she needs. Betsy has very good doctors, but sometimes I still have to be more persistent and forceful than I prefer to be in order to make sure that she gets what she needs. That is mainly more true in the ER than with Betsy's actual doctors. I have also learned to write down everything, from what is discussed at office visits, to every time a nurse comes to her room, whether it's to take her BP or give her medicine. I also write down every time Betsy has pain and include the time, how severe it is, and what activities she did that day.

Finding the Right Treatment Plan For Your Child

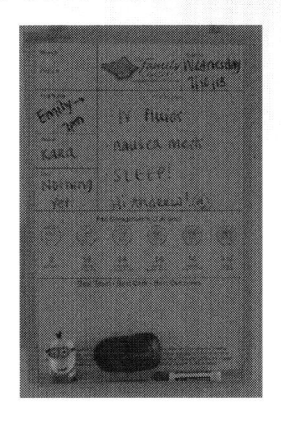

Everything is a give and take. Take the bad to get the good and try to find the right balance. But what do you do when you are no longer sure which are worse, the side effects of a drug or the problem it is supposed to solve?

When we started with CVS, a simple dose of Zofran and IV fluids was helpful. Then we progressed to needing to do Zofran, Ativan and IV fluids in combination. Doctors like to give time to see if a med works several times before changing them... so we felt very helpless as we went through the trial and error process. Then we added preventative meds option 1 (too sedating and was still frequently getting sick) then to preventative med option 2 (which he then refused to eat anything while he was on it). Then we regrouped and just go with strong abort plan for a few months until that ceases to work. When that began to fail we were forced to revisit med option 1 again (seeing the same outcomes) and the same for the previously tried second option (again with the same results). Why were we going round and round in circles?

Making choices of what side effects you can live with and which you cannot can be very difficult. Your doctor can make strong recommendations, but ultimately it's our decision as parents whether or not to agree to them, and it's our responsibility to find a way to get our child to take the medicine. It's important to be educated on the options that are out there and to participate actively in the decision-making process.

Below are some reflection questions to consider when deciding which plan best fits your child's needs:

- How often does my child get sick (daily, weekly, monthly, every 6 weeks, etc.)?
- When my child is sick and incapacitated, how long does that last (hours, days, weeks or more)?
- When my child is sick, can he or she able to still do day-to-day things?
- Can my child still read books to distract him or her?
- Focus on watching a 30 minute television show?
- Is my child in the hospital needing sedation or IV fluids?
- Is my child able to take bites of food or sips of water as needed?
- How long has this pattern been the case?
- Does this pattern impact day-to day-life?
- Can my child attend school or are they home-schooled or homebound?
- How does the child feel about this?
- How do you feel about it?
- What would be a realistic goal to set at this time?
- Can you identify triggers?
- If you can identify triggers, what changes can you make to try to avoid them?

- Have you reached out to support groups to learn what other parents are doing?
- Can you try other supportive therapies such as OT, Cognitive Behavioral Therapy, Chiropractic, dietary changes, or exercise to better reduce triggers and promote overall health?
- What is the emotional and physical impact the cycles are taking on the child and rest of the family?

For some, the pain associated with CVS is manageable, and laying low for a week means watching TV in between puking and being able to take sips of water, avoiding major dehydration. Others dehydrate in as little as an hour, no matter how much they drank the day before, like my son. Often any sip of water serves as yet another trigger to further aggravate the retching. Sound, motion, or light can do the same. It's helpful to talk to other CVS families to gauge where your child falls on the severity scale. Things you might think are helpful might actually be aggravating the cycles. Your child might need only an abort or rescue plan, requiring medication only when sick. They might require a daily preventive medication plan.

Finding what works is not a one-time process but an ongoing ever-evolving one. As our kids grow their challenges and needs change, and so will the plan that we make to help them get through the cycles. The plan that works today might not work a year from now. Documenting these changes will be your lifeline in the future. We CVS parents need to take a proactive approach in advocating for proper medical care for our children who are unable to speak for themselves. We need to work with the doctors, understanding what the probable outcomes are for the treatments that are available to us. We should always try to remember that they call it medical *practice* because of the element of the unknown.

Approaching CVS with both realistic and hopeful expectations is key to keeping your sanity. I realized early on that doctors will work with you if you work with them, knowing what to tell them and how to ask for things. Two years after my son's initial diagnosis, things are still crazy.

We are confident at this time that everything is being done for him that can be. We are doing what we can, including homeschooling, and finally getting ABA therapy to try to address the behaviors that are aggravating his condition. Do we have a cure? No. But what we do have is knowledge of what to try and a plan that is working well and bringing him comfort quicker than any other plan we have tried before.

Treating CVS, like any of the other "rare" diseases, can make you feel like you are taking a stab in the dark. Studies are limited and few understand the nature of this condition at this time. In the future, some 20 or 30 years from now this probably will change and we will know more than we do today. For now, we must ask how can we help them, who can we trust, and what we are willing to try.

We log the side effects, weigh the risks and make decisions, over and over again. We try the medications that are suggested, and we bear the burden of actually getting these meds into our children. We convince our children to give it a chance and have them take the pill or gross liquid daily. I know for us, it became a battle at times because the meds never seemed to do what we would have hoped. Our son became just as discouraged as we were and kicked back against taking anything because he was still getting sick while he was on it and had no change. This is common until you find the correct medications or treatments for your child.

It is not uncommon in the early days to continue to need emergency room care as you hash out what medicines work best. We would hear from the ER doctors that our son's CVS was not being managed properly since he was still getting sick. This can feel awful, like it's our fault. Time and time again I would explain to the hospital staff that he was only just put on this medication and it will take several months to build up in his system and work well. We were, in fact, doing everything we could do to manage his CVS. His CVS just wanted to do its own thing even though we were following our team's orders. Sometimes this process just takes time. Remember: these medications are trial and error. Reassure your child, and those around you, that together you are committed to helping ease his or her suffering.

In addition to the "traditional" medication approach, there are a variety of so called alternative or supportive therapies that also aid in reducing symptoms of CVS:

- Aromatherapy and essential oils such as peppermint, ginger and others.
- Behavioral interventions. Behavioral therapies such as desensitization, distraction, imagery, relaxation, and self-hypnosis have been shown to be effective in treating chemotherapy-induced vomiting.

Treatment Options

There are many medications that are used to treat and manage this condition. There are three main ways that medications are used: *Abortive (*to stop an episode), *supportive (*during an episode), and *prophylactic* (to keep new episodes from starting). Many of these medications are used to treat other conditions, and they are considered to be "off label" when used for cyclic vomiting. It's common for CVS children to be prescribe medications for seizures, antidepressants, and blood pressure. For more medications commonly used to treat CVS see the appendix.

Genetic Testing Leading to Better Treatment Plans? Considerations in Testing

What are functional mitochondrial disorders and what does that mean? It is not the same thing as what is commonly referred to as Mitochondrial Disease, but it is thought to be caused by the same mechanism on the cellular level. The cells are unable to maintain a proper energy supply for what the body requires. The extent of the deficiency varies, as do the factors that set the process in motion, and therefore diagnosis and treatment are very complex and requires an individual approach. This topic is far more complicated than I can explain on my own. Thankfully we are blessed to have Philippa Bridge-Cook who is an experienced CVS parent and also has a Ph.D in Medical Genetics and Microbiology from the University of Toronto. She shared her experience with her daughter's CVS. Both of us had the pleasure of interviewing Dr. Richard Boles, to learn more about this area to be able to share with our fellow CVS parents.

Philippa's Path: Mom and Science Combine
Philippa Bridge-Cook, PhD

Before I even wake up fully, my ears register the sound of my twelve year old daughter throwing up. It is such a familiar middle of the night sound for me that it has ceased to be alarming. She has been throwing up on a regular basis since she was 2 years old, in episodes that come and go, usually lasting one to two days. The vomiting that comes with these episodes is violent, frequent, and often accompanied by severe abdominal pain. Without medication, she will vomit every 10 to 15 minutes for hours; luckily, for the last few years, we've sometimes been able to successfully treat these episodes with medication.

Sometimes her episodes last longer, like one recent very bad episode where she was sick for six days on and off. At times during that episode the vomiting was controlled by medication, but not always. When her medication didn't work, she would lie on the bathroom floor and moan, and say "Mommy, help me," or worse, "Mommy, I can't live." We have been told that the medications we give her—prescription Zofran, over the counter dimenhydrate (Dramamine), and Tylenol and Advil—are the only options, and that there's nothing else we can do. But when I see her suffering, I have to believe that there must be something more that can be done, because nobody should suffer like that, especially not a child.

When she was younger, the episodes would come every month or two. She is my oldest child, and for a long time I assumed she was just very susceptible to getting stomach flu, and that she was severely affected every time she got a stomach virus. As my other two children got older, and I realized how unusual the severity of her vomiting was, and the frequency of her episodes increased, I started to suspect it was something bigger than just the stomach flu. I mentioned my concerns to her doctor, and he agreed, and suggested it might be Cyclic Vomiting Syndrome.

Cyclic vomiting syndrome, or CVS, is a poorly understood, and under recognized disorder. Although it was originally thought to be a pediatric disorder, it is now known that it can occur in all ages, and that it is more common than previously thought. It is characterized by episodes of severe nausea and vomiting that alternate with periods with no symptoms. Some patients with CVS have symptoms in addition to nausea and vomiting during episodes such as headache, dizziness, fever, sensitivity to light, and diarrhea. For each individual with CVS, the episodes are similar to each other: they generally start at the same time of day, include the same symptoms, and last the same length of time. For my daughter, she always started vomiting in the middle of the night or early in the morning, it lasted about a day, and occurred every month or two. As she gets older, everything about her episodes has become less predictable. They have sometimes lasted longer, or clustered in groups where she can have one episode per week for three weeks, then nothing for three months. CVS is thought to be a part of the migraine spectrum, and sometimes patients are able to identify things that trigger episodes such as certain foods, illnesses, cyclical hormone changes, stress, or fatigue.

Cyclic vomiting syndrome is difficult to diagnose, because there is no specific test for the disorder. Therefore, it must be diagnosed by excluding all other possible reasons for the vomiting and other symptoms. My daughter was referred to a gastroenterologist and an endocrinologist. In addition to her episodes of vomiting, she is very small for her age. After a workup by both doctors, they couldn't find any reason for her vomiting or her small size. Her gastroenterologist was reluctant to offer any diagnosis at all, even when I asked about CVS.

Because there is no physiological defect that with CVS can be measured by the medical tests we have currently, many times patients are told that their problems must be "in their head," or just caused by anxiety, depression, or other mental health problems. Similar attitudes are faced by patients with many other functional disorders, which are diseases where no specific defects can be observed by medical tests. Functional disorders include fibromyalgia, irritable bowel syndrome, migraines, chronic fatigue syndrome, complex regional pain syndrome, and restless legs syndrome. It is short-sighted and insulting to patients to conclude that their problems are not real just because current diagnostic tests can't detect a defect, and in many cases disbelief or dismissal by medical professionals leads to long diagnostic delays, during which time the patient suffers needlessly without treatment.

My daughter was faced with a version of this attitude, when for a time her gastroenterologist seemed to question repeatedly whether she might have anorexia or bulimia. The concern is legitimate, and it is important to rule out the possibility; however, the issue seemed to come up over and over again for us despite our answers. My daughter was asked if she ever didn't eat because she was worried about getting fat, and she looked very surprised, because she's worried about the exact opposite—she would love to be bigger. Clearly she doesn't have bulimia, when she is waking up in the middle of the night and vomiting in her bed, and writhing in pain on the bathroom floor. Sometimes it gets very frustrating when doctors don't seem to listen to and hear the answers that they are being given, because they have other ideas that conflict with what you are saying.

We were lucky, because my daughter's pediatrician mentioned CVS as a possibility very early on. Otherwise I don't think we would have any idea what her diagnosis might be, because her gastroenterologist was content to just rule things out based on test results, and not offer any opinion on what the problem actually is. It has been beneficial for us to have what we think is a likely possibility for a diagnosis, because it has allowed us to figure out strategies for helping her, including trying to avoid her triggers. The medication that was prescribed by her pediatrician is very useful for helping to manage her episodes when they do happen, although it isn't as much of a complete solution as I would like, and I am still searching for additional treatments that may help. However, her episodes are less debilitating than they used to be thanks to the medication, and overall she is thriving despite her illness: in between episodes she is a happy, healthy twelve-year-old who loves figure skating, soccer, *Glee*, and texting her friends.

Although it has long been thought to be related to migraines, many sources state that the cause of cyclic vomiting syndrome is not known. Mechanisms that may be involved include episodic dysautonomia (malfunction of the autonomic nervous system that can result in a variety of symptoms), mitochondrial DNA mutations that cause deficits in cellular energy production, and heightened stress response that causes vomiting. However, there is mounting evidence for the role of mitochondrial dysfunction in the pathogenesis of this disease, a fact that is not often understood by the average practicing gastroenterologist. The connection to mitochondrial dysfunction has important implications for effective treatment of Cyclic Vomiting Syndrome.

Mitochondria are small organelles within the cell responsible for energy production and other critical functions. Because of these crucial functions, Dr. Richard Boles, Director of the Metabolic and Mitochondrial Disorders Clinic at Children's Hospital Los Angeles, explains that "30 years or so ago, many scientists couldn't believe that mitochondrial disease could exist, because how does the organism survive?" However, mitochondrial dysfunction plays a role in many diseases, including CVS, and according to Dr. Boles:

"These are partial defects. Mitochondrial dysfunction doesn't really cause anything, what it does is predisposes towards seemingly everything. It's one of many risk factors in multifactorial disease. It can predispose towards epilepsy, chronic fatigue, and even autism, but it doesn't do it alone. It does it in combination with other factors, which is why in a family with a single mutation going through the family, everyone in the family is affected in a different way. Because it predisposes for disease throughout the entire system."

DNA mutations that affect mitochondrial function can occur in the DNA that is found in the nucleus of the cell (genomic DNA), or they can occur in the DNA that is found within the mitochondria themselves. Mitochondrial DNA is inherited differently than nuclear DNA. Most people are familiar with the inheritance of nuclear DNA, in which we have two copies of every gene, and we inherit one copy from each of our parents. However, mitochondrial DNA is inherited exclusively through the mother; therefore, mutations that affect the mitochondrial DNA can be traced through the maternal lineage of a family.

A possible relationship between Cyclic Vomiting Syndrome and mitochondrial dysfunction was suggested by the finding that in some families, CVS was maternally inherited. Mitochondrial DNA mutations and deletions have been reported in patients with CVS, and disease manifestations of mitochondrial dysfunction have been found in the maternal relatives of patients with CVS. In other words, conditions such as migraines, irritable bowel syndrome, depression, and hypothyroidism, are often found in the maternal relatives of patients with CVS.

Mitochondrial DNA mutations don't cause CVS directly, in the way that a DNA mutation causes cystic fibrosis, for example. In some patients, mitochondrial dysfunction plays a greater role in the causation of their disease, and in other patients, it may be less of a factor. Dr. Boles explains: "In some cases it's a clear mitochondrial disorder, they have multiple other manifestations and it drives the disease. However, in most patients, it is one of many factors in disease pathogenesis." Patients with classical mitochondrial disorders have disease manifestations such as muscle weakness, neurological problems, autism, developmental delays, gastrointestinal disorders, and autonomic dysfunction. Some patients with CVS have these other disease manifestations, and some have only CVS symptoms.

As with many diseases, understanding at least some of the cause of CVS has allowed for the development of treatments tailored towards fixing the root cause. Co-enzyme Q10 and L-carnitine are two dietary supplements that have been used to treat a wide variety of conditions.

Both supplements may be able to assist the mitochondria with energy production and thus, help compensate for mitochondrial dysfunction. A retrospective chart review study found that using these two supplements, along with a dietary protocol of fasting avoidance (having three meals and three snacks per day), was able to decrease the occurrence of, or completely resolve, the CVS episodes in some patients. In those patients who didn't respond to treatment with supplements alone, the addition of amitriptyline or cyproheptadine, two medications that have been used for prevention of CVS episodes, helped to resolve or decrease the episodes. Treatment with the cofactors alone was well tolerated with no side effects, and treatment with cofactors plus amitriptyline or cyproheptadine was tolerated by most patients. Therefore effective treatment for prevention of CVS episodes does exist, although it may not be widely employed by most gastroenterologists.

My daughter is currently trying to treat her CVS with the combination of co-enzyme Q10 and L-carnitine. So far she hasn't experienced any side-effects, and over the next few months we will see if she experiences a decrease or even a complete cessation of her episodes. My hope for her is that she won't have to choose between missing out on a fun night with her friends, and being able to be functional for the rest of the weekend. Maybe she can be like every other teenager and go to a sleepover, and just be grumpy the next day, instead of spending the next day vomiting and lying on the bathroom floor in pain.[2]

Our Experience with Genetic Testing

As Philippa Bridge-Cook noted previously, the genetic connection is a rapidly growing and often misunderstood. The first time I mentioned genetic testing for my son, I was not taken very seriously. I researched mitochondrial disorders further and laid out the family history of who had what, staying up late for weeks in preparation, during the six months wait for this appointment. We finally got in

---

[2] http://www.hormonesmatter.com/cyclic-vomiting-syndrome-mitochondrial-dysfunction/

there and…….nothing. I left perplexed and feeling lost. Again we were told that there were a variety of reasons his lab results could have come out the way they had. Again I asked about the notion of functional mitochondrial disorders and again I was met with blank stares. These were respected doctors from Boston. Why did they not share my enthusiasm and desperation to look further into this and find a better treatment plan for my son? For the answer to this I contacted Dr. Richard Boles, MD, who has been a great resource for the CVS community for several years.

The first question I had for Dr. Boles was why did many genetic professionals not offer any assistance and look at me like I was crazy. Dr. Boles explained to me that it was more a matter of the vantage point that many western medical professionals take. In our current system, medical professionals often are grouped by specialty and often do not take enough time to consider how everything is related. In his presentations that he gave for the Cyclic Vomiting Association conference this past June, he presented an image of several blindfolded people touching an elephant to try to figure what the animal was. Each guessed what it was by the small piece of the elephant they were touching. What they each were missing was the bigger picture. This is a good analogy for what many medical professionals are doing now.

Dr. Boles and others like him feel it is important to take a step back and look at the whole person — what other conditions the person suffers from, and how they could be related. For example, my son with CVS also has autism, anxiety, and is suspected to have learning disabilities as well. Could these all be connected? Could a problem lie in the genetic material previously described? Could a lack of proper energy supply be the root of all of these conditions? A holistic approach asks these sorts of questions.

How should we look into energy related issues with genetic testing? Dr. Boles explained to me that most genetic testing is like walking in a library and merely scanning the titles of the books— you often do not know enough about a book's content from such limited information.

Making decisions about how the genes work from the limited information made available by other methods of genetic testing is like that. The testing that Dr. Boles assisted in creating looks at the genes on the page-by-page level to see what information is contained in each book rather than other tests that would just look at the covers. That sounds like a lot of information to process, and it is, but we have to start somewhere if we really want to understand the mechanism of Cyclic Vomiting and other conditions like it.

Currently Dr. Boles and his team are diligently working and believe they have discovered at least two genes that they suspect are related to CVS. This knowledge is changing the ways in which treatments are being targeted, and it explains why in some cases people respond better to one plan as opposed to another. CVS is tied into both genetic and environmental factors. Complexity arises with the fact that CVS sufferers often have a variety of triggers, which often entails that any treatment plan must be very individualized. There is no one-size-fits-all treatment plan for CVS. The key, as you have seen in each of the stories included in this book, is how CVS sufferers tuned into the triggers and were able to contain the CVS.

As life changes, so will the CVS. Some years it will remain dormant, other years it will strongly make its presence known. That's how it has been experienced in my family for the last three generations. CVS can be very challenging to predict what it will do. Even within my family each generation has its own presentation different from the rest. We are working with genetic teams to see if we can find any correlation with my mother, my son and myself and the course that each's CVS is taking. My mother has moved into hemleplegic migraines, while I only have an attack when I am under stress or in need of sleep. Which way Andrew will go is anyone's guess. I can hope and pray that he takes after me and it will decrease over time. I know that the environmental stressors are often just as an important piece of the puzzle as the genetics are. I pray that with the knowledge of how CVS has presented in our family we are better able to help future generations have a chance of managing it better.

Sarina's Path: Finding the Right Plan More Than Once
Chandra Wilson

The worst part about Cyclic Vomiting Syndrome is that the cycles can come in cycles. As mentioned before, there can be an extended period of time without episodes, then, for one reason or another, they unexpectedly return. I am a CVS parent and I am also known for playing Dr. Miranda Bailey on ABC's *Grey's Anatomy*.

My daughter Sarina began CVS cycles in November of her 11th grade year and went on an 11 month journey of trial and error treatments before finding the right medicine combination that halted her episodes for almost two years. That 11 months consisted of monthly hospital stays coinciding with her menstrual cycles, grueling nausea and abdominal migraine episodes, bilious emesis almost immediately, being transferred from GI to gynecology to medical genetics, having an exploratory laparotomy, and seeing a 25 pound weight loss. CVS was finally the official diagnosis as a result of mitochondrial disease, but who knew that the two years would only be a break instead of a full remission? She graduated high school, went on to college, then noticed her energy level changing towards the end of her freshman year. She had two (not full and no hospital) episodes of CVS in May and June at the end of the term that did not coincide with her menses, so she came home and conserved her body's energy that summer.

Within two months of returning to college for her sophomore year, she began her first of 19 consecutive months of hospitalizations with severe CVS episodes. Her trigger was more constipation-related this time, and she gained weight instead of losing it. She had to take three semesters of medical withdrawals as a result of all of the hospital stays, eventually moving back home from the dorms. During this first full year, no significant change was made to her medications. After many team meetings and an extensive amount of my charting her episodes, her medical team started looking at neurological triggers to nausea and vomiting instead of abdominal ones. She had to start thinking "out of the box" and incorporated biofeedback therapy and weekly acupuncture as well. This set of relapses showed the medical team the progressive nature of her disease and the need to have to change her treatment regimen if necessary. She finally became well enough to re-enroll in school without having absences, but even Sarina is only guardedly optimistic about this stage of her break from episodes.

Fernanda's Path: Searching for Other Parents

When our own local doctors are unsuccessful in finding the best treatment plan for our child, many of us now take to the internet. We search out worldwide support groups in hopes of finding new ideas to help ease the suffering of our children. That's exactly what Fernanda did. She was on the Cyclic Vomiting Association Facebook page when she noticed my posts about my son. Her daughter was similar in age, displaying similar symptoms and her doctors were just a stumped as far as what to do. She reached out to me and became my first CVS friend. Many a night we would converse with each other about the emotional toll of CVS and what treatments were working or not working, both of us desperate to find a better plan for our child.

Time difference did not matter; our kids seemed to be on the same pattern and were in the hospital at the same time often. This came in handy when you need encouragement at 2 a.m. with a sick child. I was in New Hampshire USA and she was in Brazil but that did not matter. Through this friendship that we formed we learned what a variety of medicines were called in other countries. A key resource to remember, in addition to the doctors that we seek out, is the resource of our fellow parents who are dealing with this day in and day out as well.

There are many reasons for people to join a support group. Of those I spoke to, the biggest blessing to come from them was validation. Sure, from time to time there are differences of opinions and hurt feelings, but overall they all expressed the tremendous value in them. With some many internet and conference call options and the sheer number of groups out there, you are bound to connect with at least one group. It's very likely that you would find a group that fits your values, whose members have similar experiences and concerns as you. You might find it helpful to give back and mentor someone just starting out in the process, or walk alongside a fellow parent.

> I have seen many great things as a result of the CVSA Facebook page. We have reached thousands of people, giving them hope. It's been amazing to see someone go through the process of discovery, when they realize there are many people out there who share this condition. Facebook has given CVSA the ability to reach so many more people in a very inexpensive manner. Its great to see some living in the same geographic area to actually connect and support one another. For the rest of us there are the AccuConference support calls. While I hate seeing others go through this, it's helpful to me that there are so many others out there that also share this.
>
> Patti Mahler Administrator to CVSA/USA Facebook Online Support Group

I've participated in numerous groups and asked others why they felt the support groups were so important. Karen Anderson shares that "a support group would be great. At least then you would be able to talk to someone who understands what you and your child is going through." Sasha Kelly confirms this as well. She felt that "a good support group is invaluable" and goes on to say that "support stops you from feeling isolated and alone, it provides information and insight that no doctor (or non suffer) can provide".

Leslie Laubrick describes it as "take absolute loneliness and cover yourself with no answers, rejected by professionals and add in disbelief by everyone else. YES it is essential to have a support group". Jessica Johnson shares: "people who see my child healthy just assume that it is not as bad as I make it sound. They do not understand how hard it is to see your otherwise healthy child vomiting every few minutes for hours." We seem to get each other very quickly. We tend to embrace each other just as quickly.

Adrienne in her blog notes how parents of child with an illness or disability connect to each other in a unique way. She explains how

"if you come to us and say, *hey, I'm in trouble, I have a kid with problems and I think I belong in your club*, we will gather you into our circle so fast you won't quite know what hit you. We will listen to you cry and we won't tell you to stop. We won't tell you to be strong because we know you are being exactly as strong as you can be. We know that your need is deep and that you can't handle this, even as you are in the midst of handling it."

Together we can share experiences, offer suggestions, lend an ear and validate each other. This is an absolutely priceless gift that only a fellow parent can give.

Angie's Path: Facebook Support Group
Angie Crooks

My name is Angie and I suffer with CVS. I've had CVS since I was 14 years old, which is 22 years. I was diagnosed in 2008. I was sitting at home on one day thinking what I can do to help people with CVS even when I'm stuck at home unwell and Facebook was the answer. I started a Facebook group called 'Cyclic Vomiting Syndrome (CVS) Support Group' with the intention of using it for supporting people with CVS, adding CVS information and raising awareness.

The group really took off and soon we had hundreds of members from all over the world. The members love the group and are so happy to find people who can relate to what they or their loved one has. We talk about all kinds of subjects like symptoms, medication, feelings, medical staff, hospital visits, raising awareness and lots more. We also offer support to each other when times are rough which has proved valuable to many members. We share stories of sadness and joy and we help one another daily. It's amazing. I'm also an administrator of the Facebook sister page called 'Cyclic Vomiting Syndrome' which has over 2000 likes from people worldwide. This is an information page where I add information, news article links, stories, posters and lots more.

Being an administrator of a large group can be challenging sometimes but it is such a pleasure to do. I can help people like myself that suffer with CVS even when I can't leave the house and that's a blessing because I still feel like I'm doing something even when I'm stuck in bed. I try to add things to the group and page when I'm well enough to and try to log on daily to add members and check posts, but sometimes this can be hard to do when I'm unwell almost daily.

Finding Help Close to Home and Far Away

It was explained to us that it is important to have someone local who can advocate for you with the local teams who will be providing treatment be it in the emergency rooms or direct admit to pediatric floors. Where the specialists like Dr. Li or another experienced physician come in is teaching us as parents what to do and how to advocate for our kids to get the care they need. Specialists are good also for complex cases once all other treatments plans have failed.

We must at the same time remember the importance of establishing a working relationship close to home as well. We need to remember that a specialist from a far off place is just another doctor whom the local physicians do not know. They tend to respond better to someone they have worked with and have an established relationship with and value their opinion. Doctors can be territorial in thinking they have all the answers and do not need to be told what to do by unknown doctors. Many doctors are able to show great professionalism regarding following another doctor treatment plan while others do not. Some are more cautious because they are the ones responsible for the care of the patient and are not willing to use a protocol they are unfamiliar with even if it is documented.

This balance can be the challenge for working with CVS kids and parents who are advocating for them. Personally I have found letting them jump through their hoops works best. I have laughed at one for suggesting oral meds were the answer even though he read through my son's extensive history on file in that particular emergency room. I typically keep a good composure but I had been up for almost 26 hours at that point. Eventually he did come around and ordered the IV, once he saw the bloody vomit. We had a treatment letter from someone who works at that hospital, who was easily accessible to their staff if there were any questions about it. After a while both the nursing staff and the majority of treating physicians were well aware of his plan and relied on what I said was his current plan for determining what his medical care would be.

No one medical professional will be able to solve this for us, but with a team approach we are able to improve our kids' quality of life and care when they are sick. We are grateful for all that we have. The quality of life that my son has gained from having both better trigger control and treatment options is tremendous. What is important is to develop a positive outlook on it and to appreciate each baby step as they come. CVS will be part of their lives, we can't change that…. what we do is reassure them that we as caregivers will be there to help. We will continue to seek out answers and better ways to help.

Where in the World: Best Places for Childhood CVS

The Cyclic Vomiting Syndrome Program at Children's Hospital of Wisconsin is the largest program of its kind in the U.S. with experts who treat children experiencing severe, recurrent vomiting episodes. This is thanks to Dr. B U K Li, mentioned earlier, who was part of the team that formed the CVSA. There are other places and other doctors that are familiar with treating CVS. The Children's Hospital of Wisconsin, however, is the only place in the country that devotes itself to children with Cyclic Vomiting Syndrome. That being said, I am sure that this clinic must have a constant flow of patients. They also are willing to consult with other physicians to assist in the care of CVS patients.

The Cyclic Vomiting Syndrome Association offers a physician referral service to help people find someone experienced with CVS. Internet support groups are also helpful in this regard. Ask people in your group if they know of any local physicians who might be willing to speak to your local team. If you are not able to find a physician in your area that is listed or known for CVS experience, remember you can be the change the world needs. Medical schools might have brushed over the topic of children and rare variants of migraines, such as CVS, and may have never really gone into what it looks like. Just because your doctor has not learned much about CVS doesn't mean it's not real. Rare diseases are not well known, even among medical professionals. This is a fact that is not likely to change anytime soon. That being said, physicians have on-the-job training and often learn more about conditions when they are faced with them in their actual practice. This is where we, the parents of kids with CVS, can play an important role in helping change the perception of how the medical community views us.

We have been forming, case by case, physician by physician, a grassroots awareness about the condition. This comes when we find doctors who are young and are often more trained in teamwork mentality and are willing to seek the right treatments with us. There is a new mindset among physicians who are graduated medical school within the last 10-15 years which takes into account the whole patient and include them in the decision about their care. These physicians realize the complexity of medicine and how they are a part of a team in caring for patients. Many of them realize that they are no longer the absolute dictators of health and illness, but rather partners with their patients and a resource for parents. We need only to find the right team of professionals who are open to work WITH us and LEARN with us. The Cyclic Vomiting Syndrome Association has lists of recent research papers and studies that can easily be printed off and shared with your provider.

Riding Out the Storm of a CVS Cycle

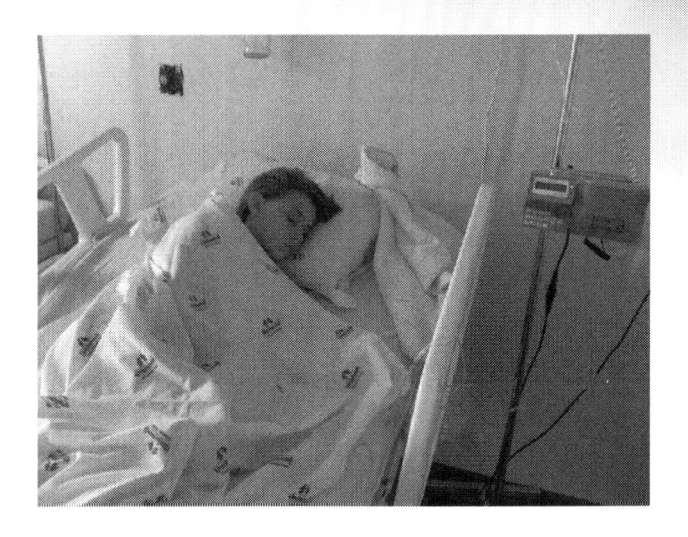

Watch, O Lord, with those who wake, or watch, or weep tonight, and give your angels charge over those who sleep. Tend to your sick ones, O Lord Christ. Rest your weary ones. Bless your dying ones. Soothe your suffering ones. Pity your afflicted ones. Shield your joyous ones. And for all your love's sake. Amen.

Saint Augustine

What a Cycle Feels Like
Karlee, age 20

Almost two years ago, I started having CVS attacks on a monthly or bi-monthly basis. It all kind of starts out of nowhere. I'm sitting on the couch, watching TV with my boyfriend, or at work, or at school. It's a sudden realization… "Oh my God, I'm going to have an attack." This is the beginning of something called the prodrome phase. Sometimes I'm lucky enough to have my emergency medication available before prodrome is over, because if I don't take it fast enough, there's no turning back. I take four or five different medications and sit, waiting.

It's a gamble because there's always the chance that I will start to throw up before they kick in. It feels like someone has punched me in my stomach. I start to sweat and shiver uncontrollably. It becomes impossible to be comfortable, no matter what position I'm in, and it gets harder to breathe. I can only think of sleep, and wanting to sleep. That is the only light at the end of the tunnel for sufferers of CVS. It feels like someone is sitting on my chest and I can't believe how cold my hands have become.

I feel the muscles in my stomach and esophagus start to spasm and I know it's too late, the medicine didn't work. The attacks are almost always typical, and mine last between 12 and 18 hours. I realize that there's nothing I can do but accept the fact that I will be very sick for the next day at least. I will not get sleep for at least 12 more hours. This is a tough realization. I always just sit and think 'why?' Did I do something to deserve this? And then it really starts. It's a bit startling at the beginning. I never know for sure how bad things are going to be. It starts violently, and I spend the first couple hours just throwing up until there's virtually nothing left. This is not like the stomach flu, and it's not like food poisoning. There is no relief. You don't get any time to recover. It's a seizure of the stomach muscles, and they will keep seizing no matter what you do.

By the time I've run out of stomach contents, I am in full swing of the attack. This is when the retching starts. With nothing coming up anymore, the stomach spasm results in a gurgling scream. I only have between 30 seconds and 2 minutes before it happens again. This is when the delirium starts. I lose my ability to differentiate between what's real and what not. I hear things, I hear people talking. I see spots and stars that float around the periphery of my vision. I close my eyes for about 10 seconds and wake up to a jolt, thinking I was asleep for hours. My mind starts to go on autopilot in an attempt to escape this new reality. If there are words anywhere in the room, I read them over and over until they become meaningless or completely change into nonsense. There's junk mail on the floor and I can make out one word. Doorbusters. ...Doobsters. Doublers. Dubsteppers. Darstraps. Stoobstars.

This is how my mind starts working. I can't grasp words and their meanings. Songs get stuck in my head until they're maddening. All the while, I'm still heaving and sweating and shaking. The vomiting doesn't stop, I keep bringing up straight stomach acid. My throat starts to burn and I've torn muscles in my stomach before that have caused me to throw up blood. I keep a drink close by so I can rinse out my mouth and attempt to save myself from the burning. My lips start to burn too, and sometimes crack because of the acid. It's only been about 3 hours.

The time gap between when I'm throwing up slowly gets longer, but the pain doesn't slow down. It feels like I swallowed a baseball covered in icy hot. I can't lay down, I can only sit up. If I feel exhausted and lay back, I immediately have to throw up again. I'm held captive in a state of semi consciousness and searing pain. This part of the attack lasts about seven or eight hours. Seven or eight hours of misery. I have to hold my head up and often nod out for a minute. Laying down causes my esophagus to burn, and I can't take any medicine for it so my only choice is sitting up. I can't feel my hands, and my arms and legs are tingling. I get bad spasms in my facial muscles and end up making contorted faces. My fingers and toes claw up and I find it hard to control them. I get heart palpitations and it feels like someone is pounding on my chest. By this point, I'm usually silently praying for death, or at least sleep. I don't receive either.

By the time I get to the last phase, I'm already weaker than I would think someone could be and still be alive. My body has cast out every liquid I had inside me and now I just have to sit and shiver. I always try to sleep by this time. It's torture, I just keep watching the clock. Any sounds or moving light distort my brain's ability to function and so I sit in silence. I lay back and only throw up about 60% of the time. I still can't roll over on my side, or move at all. But being flat takes much less energy than sitting up. I fall asleep, and open my eyes again, just hoping it's been a couple hours, and it's closer to the end of all of this. It's only been three minutes. Repeat.

This part is less predictable. it could be two hours, or it could be six or seven. I never know when the throwing up will be over, but it continually slows down. All I want is to sleep. I keep rolling through the temperatures. Hot. Cold. Hot. Cold. Sweat. Shiver. Sweat. Shiver. I start drinking water, even though I can't keep it down. It almost always ends the same way, I will go maybe up to an hour without throwing up, then I have one grand finale [usually partially through my nose] and then it's over. The pain and nausea won't be gone for another day or so, but the time for sleeping has arrived, and I'm no longer throwing up.

I spend the next day on a strict diet of Gatorade, and don't eat again until the next day after that. The time in between attacks is basically constant fear. I never know when it's going to happen. Every time I feel anything in my stomach, I start getting scared that I won't be okay. Every day is a struggle. I've been on preventative medication for almost a year now but it hasn't been entirely effective. I'm trying more options. I am willing to undergo any treatment to make my CVS go away. Anything is better than this, I promise you. Thankfully, I currently have an injection pen that I can use if I feel an attack coming on. It hasn't proven entirely effective either, but it has saved me a couple times.

But I want you to know what my life is like, currently. I'm constantly trying different medications and treatments. I haven't found anything that works yet. But this is my main focus right now. I've essentially stopped my life in order to try to get better. There's no known cause for CVS. It's just something that happens, unfortunately. It's something that's very hard to cope with. I want to know why it happens, and I want to know that there's something I can do about it. Currently, I'm powerless. I'm waiting to find something that works.

Hospitals Path: Mixed Blessing

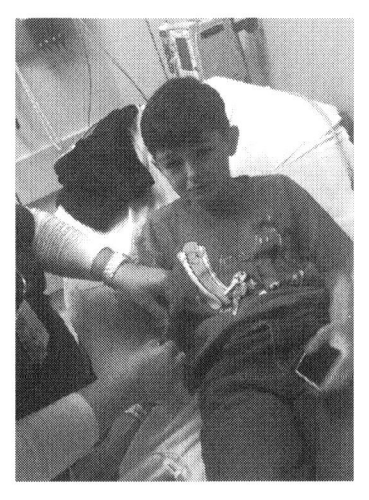

The question of when to take your child to the hospital is a common topic of concern and debate among CVS parents. Often even children with a well documented diagnosis and treatment plan in hand can be brushed off and sent home without treatment. Some physicians choose to treat only if the child is dehydrated already, while others take a proactive approach. I have had nurses ask me if CVS was even an actual diagnosis, and other times I've had one who went and looked it up while we were there in order to treat us better. The hard part is that it often all depends on who is on staff that night, and how busy the ER is, and if they are seeing a lot of gastritis. It's a big gamble when a parent brings their child to the emergency room for treatment: it could be a sweet relief, or added torture.

When I was a child my mother was explicitly told not to bring me into the hospital. The doctor's reasoning was that my mother would be better able to care for my needs at home. So she followed the doctor's advice and only would take us to the hospital in cases such as my brother's broken leg. I would ride out many cycles at home with no relief for days on end before every exciting holiday or family trip. When I was 14, a weeklong cycle resulted in my kidneys shutting down and a much needed trip to the hospital. I remember being too weak to move and telling my mom I was helping her by crushing all the ants that I saw on the car window that were not really there. I remember being carried in and having lab work done and this being literally the first time that six people did not have hold me down to do it. I remember feeling too weak, too tired and like I was slipping away.

The emergency room doctor questioned my mom — how did she know that I had not urinated in 24 hours? She knew because I had been throwing up for days and unable to drink or move on my own. They still doubted her and looked at her strangely until they got my lab results back and they realized she was correct. It took almost two days of IV fluids before my kidneys finally started to work again. It took still another two days before I was able to eat and move around. I lost about fifteen pounds in the course of the week. Without intervention I could have died. When I did get home, I had no clothes that fit and it took a while to be able to gain the weight back. This probably was the worst episode that I ever had. I would not end up in the hospital again with vomiting for another ten years. I always remembered how important it was to get IV fluids during prolonged or intense episodes or else risk having my kidneys shut down again.

There very often are times that you will find that the hospital is part of your child's treatment plan. Sometime it is as you transition from one medication to another, or in time of high unavoidable stress. I personally came quickly to realize that the most effective treatments can only be done in the hospital setting. As time goes on you might be one of the lucky ones who is able to set up home health care teams to come in and do what is needed without the trip to the hospital. Or you may be able to proactively avoid cycle by preventing them from starting.

It's not uncommon for CVS families to joke with hospital staff asking, What? no frequent flyer's club for hospital stays? There should be. If you've found yourself in the hospital once a month or more, time after time. You eventually get it down to what you need to say or do to help it go smoother. As I've shared over the last two years we've been admitted to the hospital about 22 times. The early days were nerve wracking and stressful, but by the tenth trip I think I had the routine down and it became easier. We typically end up going to the hospital around 4 a.m., which seems to be a good time because they are rarely busy then. We've also gone with newborn baby sister in tow, and always come with things we need for a lengthy stay of several days.

Hopefully you have learned that you can bypass the emergency room with the help of your Primary Care Physician. If seen in the regular office, most can then order what is known as direct admission to administer IV fluids and medications that they order. If it is after hours you may be faced with no options. In these cases it is recommended to take a proactive approach. Dr. Issenman from Canada suggests that parents meet with the head nurse while your child is well to go over plan so that they can red flag the case.[3] This proactive approach can help the process go smoother. If the staff knows ahead of time that this is a special case they may be able to work better with you. Always remember you know your child best, and you are his or her best advocate.

In the emergency room

- Keep documentation of diagnosis and treatment by your child's medical team with you. (See Keeping It Organized chapter for more information.)
- If it's a long wait ….. miss the bucket. No one likes to clean up a mess.
- If waiting in a crowded waiting room seek out a quiet dark hallway, making sure to tell staff where you will be waiting and why.
- List the reason for coming in as severe ***migraine*** instead of vomiting to dodge the "it's just a virus" comments.
- Make sure you mention the light, motion and sound sensitivity, in addition to the frequency of the vomiting.

---

[3] Cyclical Vomiting Association Conference, June 2012 WI

No matter how many times you end up there, or how good a relationship you develop with the staff, you always run the risk of the having some physician who thinks they have solved the vomiting problem and that CVS is not real during any single ER visit. Many patients are subjected to test after test by physicians who disagree with the primary diagnosis, which can be costly, as well as physically and emotionally draining. Pamela Souter has had similar experience with this as she shares how "every doctor tells me they are familiar with CVS, but nearly every doctor tries to blame the vomiting on something else!" This is response is very common and why so many opt out of the added stress during time of cycles.

Watching for Warning Signs

Ed Palmisano writes that, often as parents, "the best we can do is to become aware of these signs and we try to notice them before she does, and hope that she can start being aware of those times first." Most parents come to spot their child's warning signs and triggers. I suspect that many times parents overlook simple things in the day-to-day life that tax the child's energy. But some parents report there are no real warning signs.

Common Warning Signs

- Pallor
- Dark circles under the eyes
- Appetite change (increase or decrease)
- Mood swings and aggression
- Sore throat
- Burping or hiccups
- Changes in child's routine
- Dramatic change in energy level
- Withdrawal
- Seeking dark quiet place "bat cave"

I personally can almost always spot my son's warning signs. He gets exhausted out of nowhere and suddenly needs to sleep, or he gets easily agitated and aggressive right before an attack. His cycles typically begin during the infamous 3-5 a.m. timeframe with only a handful of daytime episodes. We know his triggers well: anything that taxes his emotional or physical energy such as going to a crowded place, going to a movie theater, or having a substitute teacher. When he was in traditional school, I always knew when something different happened at school by his behavior. I remember contacting his teachers to find out what had happened that day only to find out his teacher had not been at school that day. Who knew a different teacher for one day could derail him? But clearly it did.

My *momma sense* has evolved over the last two years. People have told me I'm being pessimistic when I've said that I knew what was coming. It is not that I want it to happen. I've just learned to read his behavior and body language. I was almost 95% correct, so I was never caught off guard or surprised, which for me made it easier to deal with. Now that he has gotten older it's changing again and we are never sure when we will be spared, when the medicines will be successful and when they will not.

I know I am not alone; I have spoken to numerous CVS parents who also know "the look" and know when to go into pretreat mode. While, again, every child is different, there are similar patterns in kids with CVS. Some kids are triggered by excitement, so you know to be prepared for holiday mishaps. Others are calendar kids who cycle every certain number of days no matter what you do. Doing our best to tune into this is a huge part of helping them.

There can be also onset signs that give you a shorter warning. Many parents have reported that their child drools or spits before the onset. Some say their child's ears turn red. Another frequent sign is the change in the pattern of their breathing, from slow to fast as they try to avoid being sick. This can happen in their sleep. Others present with more migraine-type aura such as dizziness and loss of coordination in the hours or minutes before an episode hits. Many kids are awoken out of a deep sleep in the early morning hours, so it's easy to miss the signs.

When we are able to see an episode coming, we are able to make sure we have all the medications, buckets and supplies we will need to ride out the wave of a cycle that is upon us. Pamela Souter shared her experience with this, saying that she "has to be ready, at the drop of a hat, to drop everything and tend to his emergent needs. Isaac's episodes come on quickly, with no warning, and we have around two minutes to prepare before he can no longer communicate or even hold up his own head. We have medications to give him via suppository to attempt to abort the episode, but they've never worked. He always ends up in the hospital." Some kids do not require hospitalizations, but many do.

The more you tune into your child and learn to read the behaviors, the more you are able to pretreat according to your doctor's recommendations. With CVS, there's a phrase I've heard often:

Once the horse is out of barn, there is little you can do but ride it out.

You are better off not letting it out.

I cannot stress this enough. It took me some time to understand what our doctor meant by it. As time went on, I came to see that it really was harder to stop once the cycle was in motion. Having a good abort plan was a piece of the puzzle, but what was just as important was not letting it get to that point. There are a variety of methods for this, such as lifestyle changes, diet, preventative medications or homeopathic treatments. Later on you will learn how to record and keep track of signs to help you spot trends and to be prepared the next time a cycle hits, or better yet, to be able to shut it down before it gets out of the gate.

Andrew's Path: Sweet Relief from Hospitals

At this point 99% of the emergency room staff at our local hospital know us and our case well and do not make issues of it. Remember he has sought care at this hospital over 22 times in the last 18 months or so. However, on a recent trip on Andrew's 7th birthday, the doctor choose not to look at the treatment letter we handed him nor read his extensive history on file. He walked in and said, well we will just give him oral Zofran. I laughed out loud at that. Typically, I'm a composed advocate, but I was sleep deprived and punchy on that day. He said he would not start an IV yet until he saw how the Zofran worked. I went on to explain how this was a more mild episode where he had only vomited 15 times in 2 hours which was less than usual. He then got the IV started, but was not ready to admit him yet. I then went on to explain he was about to reach the point where he vomits blood. It was the treating physician who then laughed in my face saying, oh he won't to that. And then as if on cue seconds later, up came the bloody vomit. Then he called the pediatric hospitalist who's responsible for admits down.

We have been instructed by his GI doctor to head into the hospital within an hour of onset if the abort meds fail to get it in check. This was after a history of months of having cycles every other week that would land us in the hospital for several days. We honestly did see a reduction of the length of stay and intensity once we started following this plan. We would always struggle with the decision of taking him in or not... it was a relief not to have to overthink it. The CVS UK pamphlet for nurses caring for CVS patients echoes that same idea by saying, "The faster they receive treatment the better. Delay may prolong the episode." (CVSA UK Nursing Patients with CVS)

Thankfully and finally we have been able to get better control of Andrew's CVS. Today we are able to ride more and more cycles out at home. My childhood friend Kelly West sent us a care package of essential oils to try on Andrew when he was in a cycle. We tried premade blended Pure Therapeutic Grade essential oil. I never expected them to work, but since the end of September of 2014, we have had not a single emergency room visit or hospital admission. We use a blend of ginger, peppermint, caraway seed, coriander seed, anise seed, tarrgon plan and fennel seeds blend on his belly and peppermint on a wash cloth on his head. So far it has had amazing results. We are still learning more about how this works, and have discussed it with Andrew's primary care physical and specialist before using them. I have placed resources for you to do your own research on essential oils at www.RareButNotAlone.com. Feel free to read more about them and discuss the use of them with your own medical providers.

Dana's Path: Who's to Blame?
Dana Simmons[4]

I learned early on in my sick life that if doctors can't figure out what's wrong with you, most often times, they will eventually tell you or your parents that you or your child's problems are not physical, but rather all in their heads. They make sure they tell you they tested you or your child for every physical ailment and that every test came back unremarkable, so the problem most likely is a mental manifestation.

The bottom line is that doctors would tell you either we are making ourselves sick or our parents are making us sick for attention. Unfortunately, I have read about a couple of families whose children were placed in psych wards to undergo mental treatment because as much as their parents loved their children, they thought that by believing the doctor, they were doing the right thing for their children. They believed whatever the doctor said as if it were God's own words.

Then there are the doctors who, instead of blaming the patients for making themselves sick, blame the parents for their child's suffering. If the doctors can't figure out that it's CVS, or the Abdominal Migraines causing the patients' symptoms since CVS is a diagnosis of exclusion, then some medical professionals turn to the parents and pick them for perfect candidates for Munchausen Syndrome by Proxy, which is a mental disease in which the caregiver fabricates or causes

[4] http://survivingcyclicvomitingsyndrome.blogspot.com/

symptoms of a child for attention. I know of one parent whose children were placed in foster care because they thought she was making her child sick and subsequently keeping her child out of school. The damage doctors cause by a misdiagnosis can be costly and devastating for the whole family.

I remember in the infancy of my illness, after all the tests they performed came back negative, one doctor turned to my mother and blatantly asked her if she was making me sick for attention. I remember this day clearly because my mother and I never argued with doctors until that moment. We didn't realize how destructive doctors were until my mother was blamed for making me sick after the social worker ruled out bulimia and anorexia. At that time, we respected medical providers, even revered them, but that all changed after that moment. One thing that I didn't know was that this was just the beginning of my unhealthy relationship with medical providers. It was only because I came to the realization after several meetings with doctors and nurses that they were humans just like me. They were not gods. That was when my respect for them dissipated and I considered them my equals. After all, I suffered years of abuse and neglect from several doctors and medical facilities, which made it easier for me to change my view on medical providers and the health care system.

The day they accused my mother for making me sick was the day that changed our lives forever. We learned from that day forward, that in order to get answers, we were going to have to fight for my life, and fight for a diagnosis instead of being constantly told that it was all in my head or that my mother had Munchausen Syndrome by Proxy.

I must note that while fighting for answers, and after hearing time and time again that it is all in my head, for a short while, I wondered if they were right. I questioned myself, and wondered if maybe it really was all in my head, but as quick as that idea entered my thoughts, it left even quicker. I knew what I had was real, and I knew for damn sure I wasn't making myself sick. When you get to this point, CVS sufferers, slap yourselves for even thinking that! Doctors want us to think we are crazy and that we are doing this to ourselves because it makes their jobs easier. The pain, the vomiting and the nausea were and still are so intense that I truly wouldn't wish this suffering on my worst enemy.

Again, I can't stress this enough, Cyclic Vomiting Syndrome and Abdominal Migraines are diagnoses of exclusion. What that means is that it is a diagnosis that is reached after all the necessary testing has been done and all results are negative. In addition, there are no tests to diagnose CVS or Abdominal Migraines.

That is to say, diagnosis is made only after every test has come back unremarkable, and the symptoms fits the etiology. Because of this, unfortunately, diagnosing a patient with CVS or Abdominal Migraines may take longer than five years. I have personal friends who were sufferers for decades before they were diagnosed. I was extremely lucky because it took me only a year to be diagnosed and that year felt like an eternity because of all the unexplained suffering and the looming threat of death. That is why I stress that if you think you have CVS, you must be an empowered warrior who never gives up even when all the odds are against you. After all, it's your life for which you are fighting.

It is so vital to educate people and medical professionals about CVS. Not until you find a knowledgeable doctor will you be diagnosed with Cyclic Vomiting Syndrome and/or Abdominal Migraines. Once you come to terms that it's not in your head, you can move forward. All in all, just putting a name to what's been ailing you or your loved one would truly bring a great sigh of relief, especially now that you know that all your pain and suffering was never ever all in your head.

If you would like to know more about surviving CVS as an adult, you can follow Dana's blog. Dana Simmons runs the Surviving Cyclic Vomiting Syndrome blog on blogspot.

http://survivingcyclicvomitingsyndrome.blogspot.com/

Ellie's Path: Blessing of Not Being a Frequent Flyer
Jenny Grantstrom

Sometimes I struggle with how to express my frustration and sadness with this disease. In some ways it's no big deal. It's like having asthma, something to be aware of at all times but it doesn't have to control your life. But other times, particularly when Ellie is quite sick, I want to scream and cry.

Glass Half Empty:

CVS sucks so bad! No parent wants their kid to throw-up. It's sad, it's hard to watch and you never know when it's going to happen again (an hour? a day? not for another year?). Puking is THE WORST. Last Monday night Ellie had only been asleep about an hour when she came out to the living room in tears, holding her stomach. She made it to the bathroom in just enough time. It was A LOT of vomit. Our immediate reaction was that this was not a typical CVS episode and probably the flu. Normally her episodes happen much later in the night or in the morning. Normally her episodes that involve vomit— well, the vomit is usually a lot of bile and water, not everything she had eaten that day.

Anyway, we cleaned her up, changed clothes and gave her a Zofran (anti-vomiting medicine). About an hour later she threw up again. About 45 minutes later, again. Now, if you are a parent of a little one you know that vomiting three times in one night is not easy, much less three times in less than three hours. But also, I was stumped. Why didn't the Zofran work? The Zofran has ALWAYS worked for our Eleanor. Could I give her another one? At this point she was also totally miserable, asking me if this was going to happen all night, and begging me to make it stop, so at midnight I called her pediatric gastro doctor. He said he wasn't sure why it didn't work, maybe it was the flu... Fever? Nope. Diarrhea? Nope. Been around sick people? Not that we know of. "Well," he said, "hopefully it will pass soon. As long as she is not dehydrated I'd rather she not go to the ER."

Between that midnight phone call and 2:45am Ellie vomited approximately 8-10 more times. It's like labor, the vomiting gets closer and closer together. Other things eventually happen too. Ellie goes from crying and wanting hugs to unable to even sit up to puke. I had to hold her up to vomit. She doesn't want to talk, doesn't open her eyes. And you can barely call it vomiting by the end. Her body is convulsing and some bile, a little water comes out. It goes from so sad to a little scary. At 2:45 I call the doctor back. He says, "Yes. Yes, go get her fluids." So, I wake Brian, we lay Ellie in the back seat and off she and I go to the ER.

Not surprisingly the ER people have to ask me two or three times what she has. "It's called what? And is this an official diagnosis?" The head doctor comes in and is obviously open to the diagnosis and asks me what is ER protocol for Ellie, but I have no idea because we haven't had to come to the ER since her diagnosis, so I (in my stupid and exhausted state) respond, "I think just to get her to stop vomiting?"

The nurse might have been new, he certainly was NOT talkative or a kid-person. He had a lot of trouble getting the IV in, which, once again, was absolutely so sad to watch. Poor Ellie who had barely been talking or opening her eyes was suddenly crying and telling him to stop. Another nurse came in just as this nurse got the IV in. Ugh.

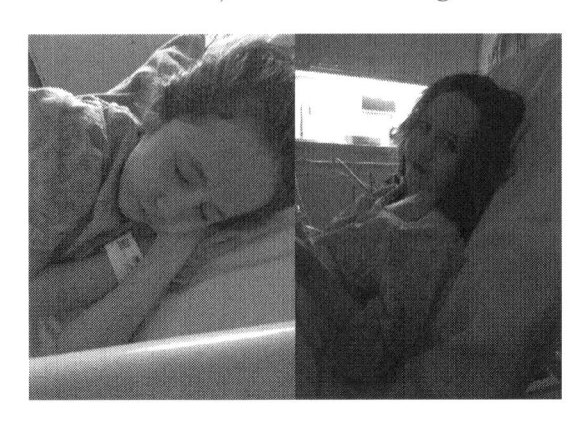

Fluids went in, another dose of Zofran in her IV and soon enough Ellie was sitting up and asking to go home. The thing was, she still didn't look good. She looked sort of yellow. She said her stomach was "3/4 good and 1/4 not good." But it had been well over an hour, maybe two, since she had last vomited, I could barely keep my eyes open (I was at almost 24 hours of awake) and I knew that if she didn't sleep—deep, restorative sleep—she wasn't going to feel better. The chances of her sleeping there were slim. It was loud, really loud. In fact, I'm pretty sure an elderly man had a terrible heart event in the little area right next to us. So, we went home. Getting out of the car she asked to be carried (not like her) then when we got into the foyer of our building she began crying and started vomiting all the water and the two saltines she had at the ER.

Because she is a total sweetheart, she immediately began apologizing in-between her hurling: "I'm so sorry Mommy! I swear I thought I was all better at the hospital!" MORE MOMMY HEARTBREAK! And here is where I had my first full blown, 100% anxiety attack since the last time I flew on a plane... my skin started getting tingly and hot, I felt light-headed, I felt I could faint, or maybe I wanted to faint... it just hit me like a ton of bricks...Her medicine didn't work. Her medicine didn't work. The ER fluids didn't work. Oh my God, what if she is going to be one of the poor souls I've read about online, who can't stop throwing up for days at a time? Brian was awake now helping us. I told him I was having a panic attack and I needed to sleep for a few hours. Ellie asked me to stay by her. I told her I just needed two hours and then I'd be back. She agreed. I went into our room and cried and cried and cried. CVS Sucks.

It passed. Ellie slept for about an hour and 45 minutes and that helped. She slept a little bit here and there throughout the day but no more puking. Then that night she was up a LOT of the night with terrible pain in her lower stomach. She would snooze for 10-20 minutes and then cry out and call for me, "Mommy? It hurts! It hurts so bad!" And then sleep for a bit and then cry out again. That went on for about three hours. I began wondering about her appendix or a UTI or a blockage in her intestines. Who has that much pain without something else going on?

The next day (day three) the pains slowed down and by 3 p.m. we went for a walk. Then the doctor called and said she should go to hospital for urine testing and x-rays to make sure the pain is nothing more than CVS. At 5 p.m. we dropped Colin off at our loving, generous, wonderful, sweet, kind, helpful cousin's house and went to do those tests. At 7 p.m. we picked up one very happy little Colin and went home for bed for everyone.

Glass Half Full:

But, as far as we know, we are not one of the poor families who are in and out of the ER or hospitalized on a regular basis. Going through last week gives me so much more appreciation for the families who haven't found medicine to stop the vomiting.

I. CAN. NOT. IMAGINE.

I really can't. Personally, I can't stand throwing up once or twice. I literally dread puking. So I honestly can't imagine what it would be like to puke so much that you end up in the ER... and then to know that you will likely have to do it all over again in a month or two or three. I have spent a good amount of my time and energy in the last few days thinking, wondering and praying that this awful episode was just a fluke, spawned by the horrible stomach flu and that her body just couldn't handle it. I feel selfish saying that since now I am friends, or at least phone call/facebook/e-mail friends, with a few families who have hospital visits as a regular occurrence for their CVS kids. But, it's a selfish desire that I think we all share. Of course, of course, we all want it to end and never happen again. That's why we are in this fight together. That's why it has been so helpful and encouraging to make other CVS friends online. We ask questions, give suggestions, feel bad for each other, and know just how it feels to watch your kiddo so miserable and know that you can't make it stop.

So in many ways we are so lucky. This is not usually a life-threatening illness and it can generally be managed. Between these hard spells Ellie has a totally average, normal day-to-day existence. Normally Ellie's medicine works wonders and I'm praying that hasn't changed, but if it has, we are connected to great doctors and specialists who will try hard to figure out how to make it better. We are so lucky that Ellie, while generally a silly, squealing, whining, girly 7-year-old, can also be wicked, wicked brave and tough. She is easily the most positive person I know and bounces back into normal life with lots of smiles and hugs and a "what's next?" attitude. And we are so lucky to have so many family and friends who don't mind my scared text messages even at 3 a.m. and don't mind my LONG LONG rambling updates like this one! We are lucky to have my Mom who has a strong bond with Ellie and wants to know every detail and would drive down in a heartbeat if we really needed help. And we are lucky to have family (cousins) just around the corner who love us so well that they check on us each day during our hard times and don't hate us when we pass the flu on to their family (So, so sorry!!).

We have so much more good in our lives than struggles...but let me tell you, at 5 a.m. in the ER with your little one in such total misery—it's easy to forget that "this too shall pass."

Debra's Path: Reminder of What's At Stake
Debra Sruggs RN

I guess I'm one of the lucky ones. I suffer through CVS and I am a nurse. What I am sharing with you, you have probably already experienced or know. I have worked as a paramedic and a nurse. I have given my life to the medical field. I've also always had a bad stomach. All my stress goes there. I've never had a headache and I always tell people and my patients you get a migraine I get to puke. I did not find out until late 2013 I have CVS - 8 hospitalizations, each a week long and another week to recover in 18 months. I have never ever heard of

CVS. I even worked with failure to thrive kiddos. I worked in the Dallas Fort Worth area. I've worked with patients already admitted and ER's. When I say I've seen it all I'm pretty darn close.

The medical field is ruthless and is for a reason. They eat their own. Chew em up and spit em out. It's a cut throat profession and if you don't have a backbone, you get one quick and you can NEVER EVER EVER be wrong. Why? **Because you are dealing with lives**. A mistake often means the difference between life and death. You learn to check, double check, and triple check everything you do. More importantly you document every little thing. You dot your i's and cross your t's. Even if it seems insignificant you document it. Why? Because if it isn't documented it isn't done. So that's an explanation as to how a medical professional's mind set is groomed and trained.

Braylee's Path: Nursing Student and CVS Mom
Labreska Mckenzy

When my Braylee was first diagnosed with CVS I was in nursing school and had never heard of this. Even in all my books, I only found one small paragraph about it. She was admitted to our small little town hospital 12 times in 18 months where sometimes her stay was a day and sometimes it was up to a week. After we were able to get this under control and didn't have so many admissions with rescue meds and etc., I had been a nurse for a few years and had never had a patient with CVS. One day, right after I started a new job, I was in report and after the nurse reporting said a name, she said, "She's back with of course same thing, nausea and vomiting, asking for something for pain and it's the same ole, same ole."

I stated that I wasn't familiar with her. She told me that she comes in all the time with the same thing and just craves meds for the vomiting and pain. She said her home meds are amitriptline and Zofran. Immediately, I asked if she had CVS. She said yes, she has something like that. I began to explain that my daughter also has this and I explained what it was. None of them had heard of it. They all "changed their tune" about this girl after that.

After I came out of report, I went to the bathroom and just cried. I knew that my daughter had been talked about like that too. And she always would be as long as CVS was something that was neither taught in nursing school nor explained to the nursing staff by the physicians.

It broke my heart that she would not be taken seriously. She has been critical with abnormal labs before to the point that it caused abnormal heart rhythms and etc. But, she will slip through the cracks because she is a "regular". Anyway, I just wanted to share that. And I'm not talking about my fellow nurses... It's not really their fault. The diagnosis was dehydration. It is just ignorance and not being educated. Something needs to change.

Trinity and Andrew's Path: Hospital Bag

Sometimes your treatment plan includes a trip to the emergency room or direct admission. As you've read in most cases IV fluids and medicines are extremely beneficial. It helps to have a hospital bag packed ahead of time so you are ready go. Often receiving medical interventions can limit your attack from days to hours. Below is a list of helpful things that we have found to have ready to go. Once I had a bag ready to go at all times it took the added stress off. When your child is sick you need to conserve your energy for more important things like advocating for your child.

- Eye mask - block out bright lights
- Weighted Blanket - helps provide comfort and deep pressure to regulate and calm nervous system
- Lollipops- (Can help with blood sugar issues some children have during cycles an it changes gross taste in their mouths.)
- Money for food for caregivers (try to get 1 hot meal a day)

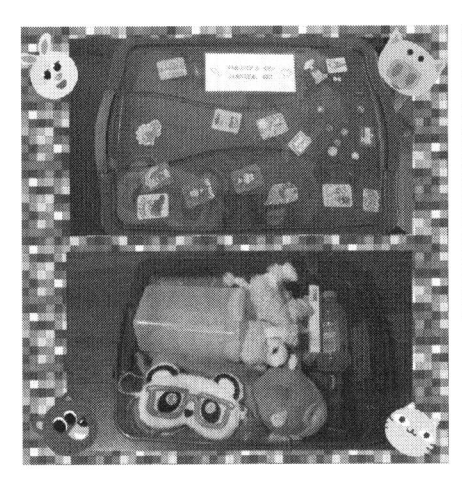

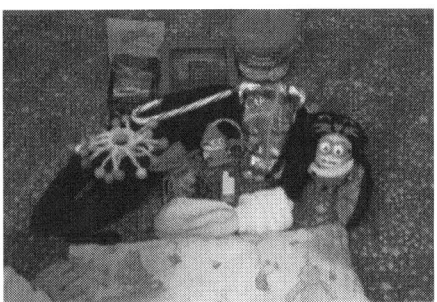

Jack's Path: Service Dogs and benefits of Pet Therapy

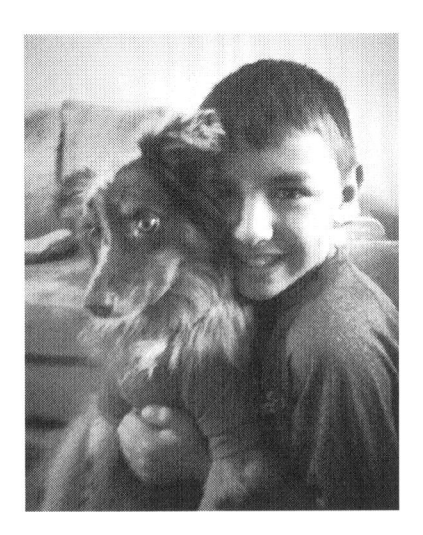

Harvey the Wonder Dog and Jack

My name is Jack, I'm 10 years old and I have CVS. I've had it for 10 years. It makes me feel "un normal." When I get sick I just can't stop throwing up and it makes me feel different. The light bothers me and it gets blurry so I cover my head.

We got this dog and he was little and nice and cute. My mom said he would tell me when I was sick and would know if something was wrong with me. He would stay around me. The first time he told me I was sick, he was being nice and laying on the couch with me and the next day I threw up. He stayed with me the whole time and sat on top of me. Sometimes he licks my face and hands when I'm going to be sick, so I can take medicine to stop my episode.

Harvey is a good dog with bad habits. He can't pass his obedience class to be a certified service dog. I still like him even though. He's fluffy, an Australian shepherd. I feel super good about Harvey in the house 'cause he's really nice and a clever dog. He makes me feel safe. I don't know what I would do without him. He makes me feel comfortable wherever we go... He just needs to stop trying to eat people's noses.

It's well-known (and scientifically proven) that interaction with a gentle, friendly pet has significant benefits. Paws for People shared with me the benefits of pet therapy.

Physical Health:

- lowers blood pressure
- releases endorphins (oxytocin) that have a calming effect
- diminishes overall physical pain
- the act of petting produces an automatic relaxation response, reducing the amount of medication some folks need

Mental Health:

- lifts spirits and lessens depression
- decreases feelings of isolation and alienation
- encourages communication
- provides comfort
- increases socialization
- reduces boredom

- lowers anxiety
- helps children overcome speech and emotional disorders
- creates motivation for the client to recover faster
- reduces loneliness

Some Other Helpful Furry Buddies

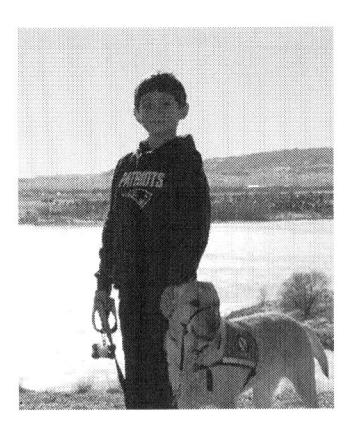

He has had a medical alert dog for six months, after several conscious coma chokings on vomit in his sleep. She can alert about an hour before an episode begins.

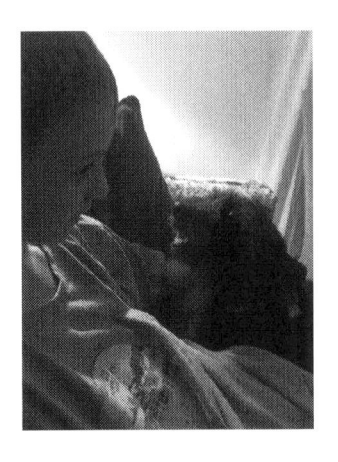

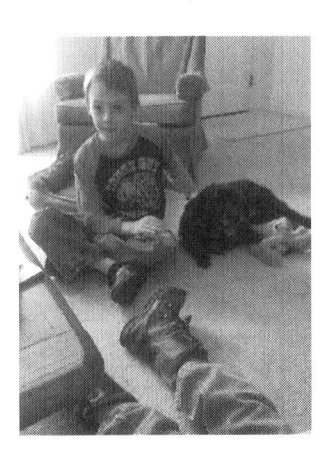

— Denise, Patrick's mom

Andrew and Betsy (grandma's dog)

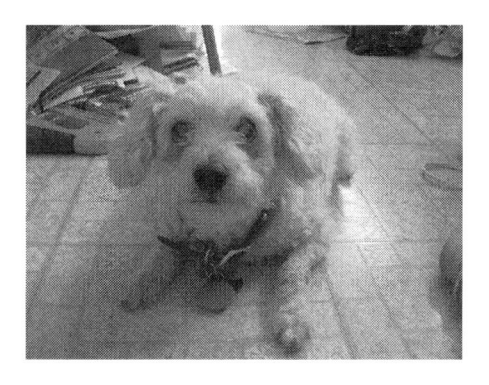

*In loving memory of Poxy.
A beloved CVS companion of over 20 years*

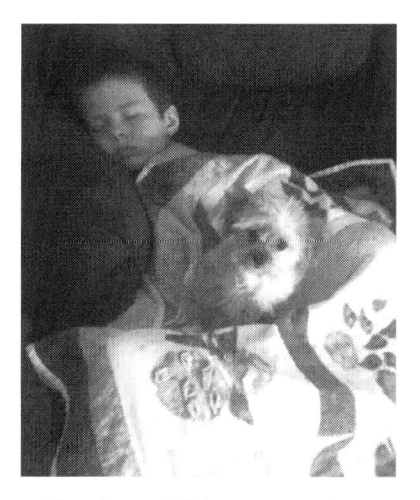

Brady and his companion

Christopher's Path: A Tragic Ending

Lisa is a CVS mom who desired to share her son's CVS journey and tragic end to help raise awareness of the need for better care and more research to be done. In 2010 her son Christopher died from complications due to CVS. Though this is a rare outcome, it still is possible nonetheless. We all should be aware of what can happen. Christopher vomited for a period of five to seven days straight every three weeks for eight years. At nine months of age he began this vomiting disorder.

He had already overcome a stroke he suffered at six months of age related to an immunization shot. His mother wonders if it was the stress that this event put on his body that set the cycles off.

They tried EVERY medication (and there were many), all which only seemed to make him worse. He only saw a reduction in the episodes with a natural diet and less chemicals. It was almost hard to believe the suffering. She shares how he used to vomit and retch to the point of producing blood, which can be common for kids with frequent cycles. Most of the time he could barely keep his head up from weakness and the acid from his vomit would literally burn holes on his face and arms. His mother shared how this was hard to explain without people believing that she was exaggerating. As CVS parents, most if not all of us, have witnessed exactly what she is describing.

His parents sought out six different university hospitals in a desperate attempt to get control of his episodes. Every doctor told them there was nothing wrong with him genetically. They did skin, muscle, and liver biopsies, and all came out showing nothing wrong with him. Yet he vomited every couple weeks for days and weeks sometimes. Keep in mind this was in 2002-2010, and the empirical guidelines for treating CVS were not published until 2007 and formally accepted in 2008. While the information of better treatments was out there, it was still new and not every physician was aware of it or familiar with implementing it.

On the days he was not in an episode he was completely healthy, which is common of children with CVS. Sadly, during one of his numerous cycles, he developed and infection that the doctors were unable to treat and it led to his untimely death less than a month before his 9th birthday. Christopher suffered for eight years and his mother continues to pray for all of the other families that live with this illness. She expressed a deep desire and hope for more studies to be done leading to a cure or until better management plans are found. She's seen it all with this illness, the highs and the lows, and unknowns. She described her son's severe case as a cancer for eight years that wouldn't go away. He has been gone three and half years and she still feels a strong need to raise awareness of this illness that might lead to one less parent suffering the loss of a child.

In Loving Memory of Christopher 9/18/01 - 8/28/10

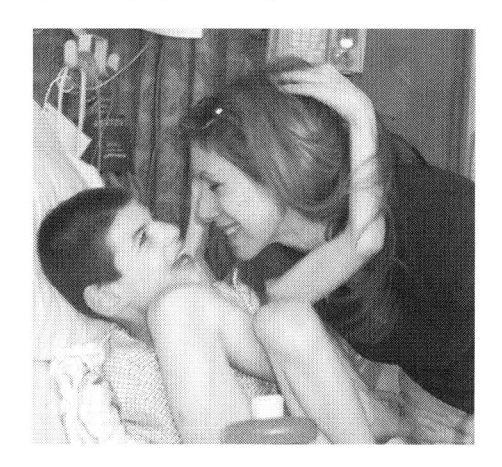

Making the Plan: Documenting Your Path

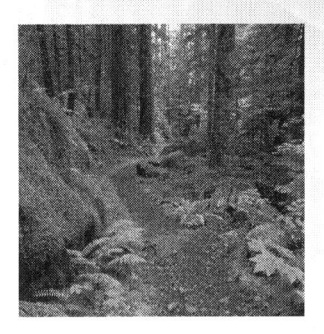

You might wonder how on earth I keep all this information straight - the doctors' contact numbers (for all the specialists), the recent office notes, what's important and what is not. What you can do? How do we keep track of it all? Is there any reason to keep a log? Many parents have so many other responsibilities, and to add managing the care of a child with Cyclic Vomiting Syndrome can feel like an additional full time job. This is where being proactive comes in handy and setting up a clear system saves you a lot of time, energy and stress. This becomes easier as the child get older, but in the early days when stress is high it is easy to become overwhelmed and forget things. It is often helpful to have a binder that contains basic info such as:

- Photo of your child when they are well and something they love to do.
- CVS Action Plan or any plan written by physician
- Cycle Log
- Home diary
- Hospital diary
- *Extreme Emesis* by Narayanan Venkatasubramani, Thangam Venkatesan and BU. K. Li.[5]

---

[5] http://practicalgastro.com/pdf/September07/Sept07VenkatasubramaniArticle.pdf

Cyclic Vomiting Action Plan SAMPLE

Green Zone	Signs and Symptoms	Treatment	How much and when
		Supplements L-carnitine COQ10 B2	
Yellow Zone	Signs and Symptoms	Treatment	How much and when
Trigger Present	Pale, dark circles under eyes, mood changes, belly pain	Take abort meds 1. 2,	
Calendar time	Appetite changes, extreme sudden exhaustion, headache	Take abort meds 1. 2.	
Red Zone (Cycle in progress)	Signs and symptoms	Treatment	
	Vomit <4 per hour Unable to sleep Unable to swallow saliva Unable to walk or talk Unable to watch TV Conscious Coma	AT ONSET give : 1. 2. Warm Shower or Bath Quiet Dark Room If abort meds are still ineffective or unable to keep in after **1 or 2 hours seek medical advice or head to ER for IV med.**	
	Vomit >4 per hour	Maintain sips of fluid and able to hold them down for 30 mins. Continue abort meds as needed till recovery phase is reached.	

*****Note: your specific plan may be different. This is merely a guideline or frame work that could be used. This would be helpful for schools to keep on file in the nurse's office.

Cycle Pattern Log (sample)

Name

Age

Cycle Dates	Cycle Length	Treatment	Trigger (if known)
June 1-3, 2012	3 days	Hospital admission	High pollen count
June 13-19, 2012	6 days	Hospital admission Brought to ER after 6 hours of uncontrolled vomiting	Last day of school
July 6, 2012	5 hours	Managed at home	Holiday

Pediatric CVS Diary

Name and Age:

Date/Time Episode Start:

Date/Time Episode End:

TOTAL Length

Warning Signs: Mood Swing Exhaustion Dark Circles

                     Headache Belly Pain

Location of Pain: Head Belly Legs Eyes

Type of Pain: Pressing Throbbing Piercing Burning

Intensity of pain   Normal 1 2 3 4 5 6 7 8 9 10 Worst

Intensity of Nausea/ Vomiting   Normal 1 2 3 4 5 6 7 8 9 10 Worst

Sensitivity of Light, Sounds   Normal 1 2 3 4 5 6 7 8 9 10 Worst

Pretreated with:
Meds taken at ONSET and how they worked:

How meds were given and did they get into child's system?
Given Orally, Rectally or IM (shot) If orally were they able to stay down at least 30 min
How long till hit dry heaves retching:

Vomit was: Food   Bile (yellow or green)   Brown (coffee grounds or Mucus)
How episode affected my normal routine:

Hours/ quality of sleep night previous:

What I ate before episodes:

Activities before episode:

Important stressful events around time of episode:

Hospital Diary

Once in the hospital the goal is rehydrate, comfort, and support until it passes. The best thing is a deep sleep which is only thing that shuts down a full cycle.

Emergency room doctor on treating:

Nurses in ER:

Pediatric doctor on duty:

Nurses on pedi floor:

VITALS

Heart rate at admission time: Blood pressure:

Admitted or treat and release:

IV meds given: How Long until effect was seen:

Number of hours slept once meds given:

Notes about med plan:

Typically med should be given together with in 15 minutes to have best sedating effect and not be spread out.

Something that helped my child:

Something I would do differently next time:

Limit nurses checking vitals.

Have no visitors until SURE of Recovery phase without rebound.

Number of times yo-yo before recovery without relapsed:

When child first spoke/ swallowed or attempted to eat food or drink:

What did my child crave?

What comforted my child?

Other Important things to remember

Choosing a Peaceful Path

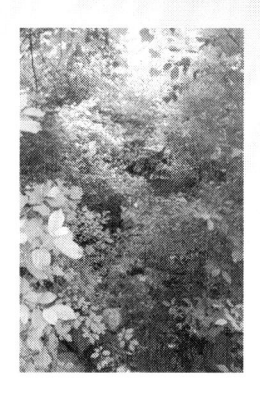

Shame abandons, encouragement believes.
Condemnation paralyzes, compassion frees.
Exasperation quits, patience prevails.
Yelling silences, communication opens up.
Blame hurts, grace heals.
Faultfinding destroys, praise builds.
Rejection loses, unconditional love wins.[6]

Finding Peace in the Storm of CVS

Is it possible to find peace while living with the storms of CVS cycles or is it something to wage a war on? Remember that many CVS kids vomit, not because of bad thing like stomach viruses, overeating, or food allergies. These kids vomit because of excitement, because of the good things that make other kids happy. Most often people think of this as a "nervous stomach," but that description is not even close to

---

[6] http://www.handsfreemama.com/2014/05/20/to-build-or-break-a-childs-spirit/

accurate. Oftentimes a person who is simply nervous will vomit and then feel better. Nervous people can be distracted by TV or something else that redirects their attention. If you are a parent of a child with cyclic vomiting, you might notice that no amount of bribing, incentive or punishment turns the vomiting off and, in fact, those distractions make it worse. Let's face it: excitement isn't easy to avoid. It's one thing to control what foods your child eats; it's quite another to manage their level of excitement!

Life is exciting! Children, by their nature, excite easily as they are filled with awe and wonder when they learn about the world around them. They love to celebrate and embrace any reason to do so. Good excitement or bad excitement, it's all the same to a CVS kid. In our house we try to focus on simple joys and ways of being content from day to day. Homeschooling has spared us the cycles that are triggered by assemblies, substitute teachers, fire drills and other seemingly harmless excitement in a child's life. Sure, you'd expect traveling to see family out of state would be one, which it is, but there are so many exciting things that happen during the day that we often overlook.

CVS children love to be happy and excited, but for some children this excitement sends their nervous systems into hyper-drive, causing a cycle of intense vomiting and sensitivity to light and motion and sound. So how can CVS kids find peace and joy in this world of excitement? In our house we teach the idea of a peaceful puke. We made the decision early on that we did not want to teach him to wage war on it.

Inner peace starts with a decision. Peace comes from within. Peaceful puking is a state of mind, knowing that this will pass. It acknowledges that a CVS child's body processes excitement differently. It's not a beast to be fought, though you and your child might feel that way at times. Emotions just are; excitement just is. How you both handle them can make a difference in the direction this illness will likely take. As cyclic vomiting parents, we need to help our children to work with their emotions and excitement, not against them. We should allow their feelings to be acknowledged and validated, thus released and less likely to become full out triggers causing things such as further anxiety or depression. I am not saying CVS is an emotional or mental disorder, but it is certainly aggravated by stress of any kind. The peaceful puker is one who, though he is fighting a battle, consciously chooses not to wage a war but rather weather the storm that he finds himself in.

At the June 2014 Cyclic Vomiting Association Conference in Milwaukee, Dr. Sally Tarbell presented a talk to help those with CVS to better understand the stress connection and offer suggestions to deal with it. Stress is physical or mental arousal triggered by the perception that something is challenging our ability to cope. Our body responds to stress in a variety of ways such as changes in muscle tension, digestion, heart rate, and blood pressure. Our attention narrows, vigilance increases, and negative thoughts and feelings can occur. Chronic stress can lead to long term harmful changes in the brain and weakening of the immune system.

Stress can be divided into two categories: controllable stress and uncontrollable. If stress is controllable, we can take action. We are able seek information, and problem solve, and modify our lifestyle with proper sleep, exercise and diet. When it comes to uncontrollable stressors we need to be focus on what we think how to frame it in helpful ways. The challenge becomes what we THINK about the stressor and what we say to ourselves. This is why the peaceful puker is a better option. When you think of war, you think of battles, fights, and pain, all of these things would feed into the body's stress response in undesirable ways.

To achieve victory, people with CVS should do the opposite, and learn to work with the body's natural responses. This approach is not about giving up. It not surrendering to CVS in a way that might be seen as a failure. Although presently there is no known cure for CVS and there may not be one in your child's lifetime, there is cause for hope. Give them the tools to pick their battles wisely and to live a full and meaningful life despite having CVS. Caregivers can help a child to become a peaceful puker, to become someone who is not shocked or emotionally defeated by yet again another cycle. Instead they encourage the child to conserve energy by not waging war on it, and it can be just another storm to weather. This way they can use what little energy they have for preparation to ride the cycle out.

My husband and I were only half joking when we said we should just do away with birthdays and holidays here. We know that's not the answer. We were reflecting on the numerous hospital admissions we've had over the last year: his birthday, the birth of his sister, his older sister's first communion, Halloween and Christmas, to name a few. We've learned to keep parties small and only to invite immediate family members, just celebrating with dinner of their choice, cake and glow balloons. Yet every birthday (of any family member, it does not have to be his) we end up in the hospital. This is so commonplace that the siblings no longer bat an eye about it.

Not all anxiety comes from negative things. It is often the positive stressor of excitement that trigger similar bodily response. I know more than once I have had to try to explain this to others. Both have an effect and require more energy from the nervous system. Both trigger the body's natural response to stress. This interconnectedness is crucial to understand that it is not a mental condition despite at one time being referred to as psychogenic vomiting. This should help people know it's not in their head in the way people think it is. Anxiety is often a trigger for CVS, and there are many people out there with anxiety who do not have CVS.

Do these kids need to learn to tolerate their excitement better? Yes. Are we sheltering our son? Not in the way that one would think. In teaching and increasing his ability to tolerate it, we need to make sure our children can succeed which may mean more breaks, or accommodations than is typical for others their age. Much depends on their tolerance level and whether parents are proactive in avoiding a cycle. As a child with CVS get older they often learn to respond better to these stressors using cognitive behavioral therapy and relaxation techniques.

A parent of a toddler or preschooler knows how hard it is to get them to bed on Christmas Eve or before the first day of school. CVS parents might fight such a battle every day. Some things will get easier the older our children get and the more positive experiences they have. If they develop quite the history of excitement puking, they will learn that this will pass, it will get better and the cycles can come and go. We've found also that they learn to have a greater appreciation for the healthy times that many take for granted.

A popular saying which is often attributed to Albert Einstein reminds us that "Everybody is a genius. But if you judge a fish by its ability to climb a tree, it will live its whole life believing that it is stupid." As a CVS parent you learn that your child processes excitement and stress differently than other kids. Expecting them to easily process these is similar to expecting a fish to climb a tree. It is possible for them to learn to improve over time and if given proper supports, but for many there will always be a level of sensitivity. What's important is the value and attention we as parents place on it. There are so many other things that they can do. We should focus on each child's strengths and what brings them joy and gets them through the storm of cycles.

Many of us are often left with the question of which came first, the chicken or the egg? Or, in our case, CVS or the anxiety? They can feed into each other, sending a child into a downward spiral until we are able to better stabilize them. We can do this by effectively managing both stressors and making sure we provide prompt relief during cycles. Anxiety is often used by others as a scapegoat for the vomiting and kids often feel that it is their weakness that is the cause of the vomiting. This can be a huge struggle for CVS parents and children.

As you will see throughout the book parents often need to try a variety of means and approaches to manage this. Some have benefited from occupational therapy for sensory integrations issues, cognitive behavioral therapy, play therapy, applied behavioral therapy pet therapy, and many more. All of these things can better support proper growth and development for every child. With CVS kids, however, when things are out of balance, you can see it in the increase of the number and severity of the cycles. Stress management can be simple, in creating an environment to reduce day to day stress.

A foundational piece of stress management is how we respond during the episodes. We have seen the best results came with a strong and fast response to treating the cycle once it hits. Having an actual plan in place and knowledge of what to try has been a tremendous help. Delaying treatment both drains a CVS patient of physical energy and adds to the already stressed condition. We have had to tweak the treatment plan over time to find what worked best for my son. Some kids will need meds, others will need to head to the hospital at first vomit. Whichever plan is recommended to you, the goal should always be to comfort your child by either reducing vomiting or pain as much as possible or promoting actual sleep in order to shut down the cycle. More suggestions from fellow parents will be shared throughout the remainder of the book.

The recognition and treatment of CVS has come a long way in just the last twenty years. With any growing field such as this, the science and documentation behind these things are ever changing as more and more discoveries are made. With this awareness that is being raised, more kids are finding the correct diagnosis and finding more relief from their unique symptoms along with validation of the reality of this identifiable medical condition.

Cristy's Path: Journey to Acceptance
Cristy Balcelles RN MSN, Exec Director of Mito Action, and author of Living Well with Mitochondrial Disease

Our purpose is to redefine what we want, what brings us real happiness, and how we can live again in spite of the CVS diagnosis. How you and your family arrive at a state of peace and acceptance about this disease depends so much on the individual. However, there are many parents, and kids, who have walked this road before us, who can offer their insight and advice. The following are "road signs" that will help you on your own CVS path.

1. *Take the Time You Need / Allow Yourself to Be Overwhelmed*
   Even if this was a diagnosis that you were expecting or had been pursuing for a long time, you still probably felt shocked

when the diagnosis was confirmed. In addition, most people have difficulty processing information and remembering any details when they receive such overwhelming news. Don't be afraid to take the time to process this new information and ask more than once for help or for information to be repeated (or better yet, written down for you to reference later).

It is normal to be overwhelmed. It is understandable when successful people who are accustomed to being able to make good decisions and control the consequences feel as if they have been punched in the stomach by surprise with the CVS diagnosis. It is "only human" to feel angry, sad, detached, depressed, afraid, or any combination of these! Even the most successful and resourceful patients, parents, and families who learn to find joy, hope, and quality of life despite the diagnosis of CVS still find themselves at rock bottom once in a while.

I say all of this not to create further despair about your life now that there is a CVS diagnosis on the table. In fact, no physician, family member, or expert can predict the future for you, your child, or your family. ALL of us have felt truly lost at one point or another during this crusade, as if they had been dropped into an alien country without knowing the language or the landmarks. Allow yourself to be overwhelmed, and give yourself the space to see beyond those feelings.

2. *Find Support in Others Who Understand*
Finding support from others who have CVS (or more broadly, special needs or chronic illness) can be the lifeline that you need when you are at the end of your rope.

3. *Recognize When You Are Overstressed*
For many, when we receive a devastating and emotional diagnosis like Cyclic Vomiting Syndrome, we instinctively feel right away that we should be "ready to fight." Today, there is a great deal of psychological theory that asserts that our society lives in a chronic state of fight or flight. We are all stressed all (or most)

of the time, and this chronic state of heightened adrenalin and arousal can actually wear us down, aging us prematurely. So how about you…are you ready to fight, flee, or freak out? Both children and adults with CVS have a tendency to become trapped in a chronic state of "fight or flight." Just because you feel tired and don't have the energy to run like a gazelle does not mean that your body is not revved up and stressed!

<u>And a few other signs just for kids</u>:

- Acting out? Tantrums, pushing, shoving, biting, yelling.
- Sleepy in inappropriate places or despite the opportunity for rest periods?
- Avoidant? Avoids eye contact, avoids talking.
- Withdrawn? Doesn't want to participate in activities—even those that he enjoys.
- Crying, tearful, anxious, begging, whining, fussing?

4. *Give Yourself Permission to Grieve*

Grieving is fundamental to acceptance of the diagnosis. Learning to live with CVS or any other chronic condition is a process. Grief is part of that process, whether you are a parent, a family member, a caregiver, a teen, or an adult patient. Often we don't allow grief to be part of the process of learning to positively cope with the diagnosis of CVS. Grieving can allow us to let go of and accept some of those fears. Grieving gives you the freedom to be sad for the loss of some of our dreams for the future.

Let me be clear: grief and acceptance are not about passively lying down and letting CVS take over your life. It is NOT giving up! Acceptance, of grief and of the diagnosis, is about dreaming new dreams, looking around for new opportunities, and seeking different perspectives from a new point of view. *Your vantage point has changed,* so we must begin taking control of the little things that make you or your child and family feel better now so that you begin to be able to consciously direct your energy in ways that make you feel well, both physically and spiritually. However, when we don't stop and allow ourselves to recognize these feelings of grief and to give ourselves (and our other family members) the time to feel sad, to be in denial, to be angry, etc., we can get stuck on an endless loop of frenetic searching.

5. *Remember to Remember*

One of the best tips I learned from an adult Mito patient is to "remember to remember" by taking advantage of the technology offered by today's computers and cell phones. Smartphones are especially great tools for managing hectic schedules by offering calendar functions with alarms and alerts that you can customize. Set the timer or calendar reminder features so that you can be automatically reminded to take or refill medicines, call for appointments, submit insurance appeals, etc. In addition, you can use the "notes" feature on smartphones to keep track of important information, such as medical record numbers, names of your medications, test results, etc.

6. *Establish Routines and Simple Rituals*

What can you realistically do every day that you enjoy? Can you have a special cup of coffee? Can you walk to the park or take a swim? Can you sit down for a moment in the afternoon or evening while you look out the window at a garden or read a book together? Can you cuddle with a pet? Begin to establish routines and simple rituals by first identifying simple things that you enjoy. Make a list—does your family look forward to fresh bread or bagels from the bakery on Sunday mornings? Often, we already have little routines that we take for granted; however, if we enjoy them, we can allow those existing routines to become sources of happiness for us. Instead of mindlessly having your coffee or going to the library, become cognizant of this activity and be very aware of the details. Peppering an otherwise stressful day with little routines and simple rituals such as a cup of tea or reading the paper can help us to feel grounded, and gives us something to look forward to even when we are feeling very sad or overwhelmed. If you're frequently in the hospital with your child, find a book to read or learn a new skill, as you might be spending a lot of time in a quiet dark place comforting your child.

7. *Become Empowered by Knowledge*
You cannot feel in control when you don't understand what's happening. Parents, you may be watching your child suffer, fail to gain weight, have confusing or erratic symptoms, and be exhausted, and no matter what you do, sometimes you cannot make it better. You will be able to put yourself in the driver's seat more often, and you will be more confident in yourself as an advocate (for yourself or for your child) when you are armed with knowledge. Knowledge is empowering. Understanding the nuances of your diagnosis and your symptoms allows you to plan better and prioritize your medical needs. You can tease out what's most threatening in your own set of symptoms when you understand what's happening in your body where an energy metabolism defect is present.

8. *Learn to See Your Child Beyond the Diagnosis*
"This is what I have, but it is not who I am."

—Teen Mito "survivor"

Our next step in learning to live with CVS or Mito is to make a conscious choice: "I am willing to accept the challenges and the pain that I might face because of my/my child's diagnosis, but we will live and be happy anyway." Here's the important distinction. *Cyclic Vomiting Syndrome is something that you have; it's not who you are.*

9. *Choose your Friends Wisely*
Have you heard of a circle of trust? There is a circle of trust, described by experts, that we unconsciously project onto the people around us. In the same manner that we are learning to dream new dreams and redefine our view of success and happiness, we are also going to benefit from being consciously choosy about the people who we turn to in need and those whom we

let in to our "circle of trust." The joy of this is that you can choose who you allow in! Again, these choices put us back in the driver's seat and give us much needed feelings of control. Perhaps there were friends who let you down but others who stepped up when you didn't expect it. Take note of this and be willing to share your anxiety, fears, or anger with the people who you can trust. On the other hand, for others, don't give them the opportunity to let you down! Choose how you relay information to them so that you are ultimately protecting yourself and your own attitude.

10. *Learn to Balance the Energy Budget*

One of the most important lessons that any caregiver or patient with mitochondrial disease can learn is energy budgeting. Did you know that Earth has an energy budget? In order to stay in a constant state of balance, or equilibrium, the physical energy expenditures must be equal to or less than incoming energy transfers. In other words, the sum of the losses should be the same as the sum of the gains. Without disruption, this equilibrium happens naturally. However, emissions, greenhouse gases, and changes made by man to the earth's surface can significantly alter the energy budget of the world!

We can extend this analogy to life with a mitochondrial disease and/or CVS. Our bodies have a similar system that needs to be in proper balance to function as it should. It is like operating with a "low battery," but this doesn't mean that a child is just tired; it means that many areas of her body will suffer from the lack of energy or power that she needs.

Adapting Outings for A CVS Child
Melissa Knight

Just because your child has a diagnosis of CVS does not mean that he or she cannot participate in fun activities. Adapting the outings or activities is a must. Depending on your child's triggers, normal day events such as going to the grocery store, playing with friends outside, and getting ready to get into the car, can trigger a CVS event. My daughter can start her vomiting cycle due to normal activities that cause her to become excited. I have learned that telling her plans too far in advance is not beneficial. I adapt by getting everything ready until we are five minutes from leaving and then I tell her where we are going.

Long car rides are also a trigger for her as well. By a long car ride, I mean anything over twenty minutes. For longer trips, it is sometimes necessary to pre-treat with medication prior to getting into the car and other times, I just adapt as we go. I always find it beneficial to sit her in the middle of the car where she can focus straight ahead. Also, having cool air by an open window helps. If she gets over heated, an abdominal migraine is right around the corner. I listen to her and if she tells me she needs me to pull over, I pull over. I can tell by her skin color that it is time to take a rest.

We have adapted trips for her as well. Last year, before I knew a lot about CVS and my daughter's triggers, we planned a weekend trip with some friends. The kids had a long day scheduled out on a boat, followed by swimming, riding bikes, and a bonfire. My daughter was only able to be on the boat for about a half hour until she was overheated. We had to be dropped off at the dock and cool water bottles were placed all over her neck and forehead. She had to go lay down. Later that night, we met everyone for the bike riding and bonfire. After being there for about an hour, my daughter starting throwing up and screaming she needed to go lay down. Once again, her face was beat red. I was not aware that exhaustion, overheating, and lack of adequate hydration could trigger her episodes. We went back to camp and I cooled her off and got her into bed.

With experience comes proper planning. My daughter loves boat rides, swimming, and playing on the playground, just as much as any other four-year-old does. I still allow her to have a childhood. It is adapted though. Now, boat trips are no more than 30 minutes at a time. She is properly hydrated and I put a baby pool on the boat for her to cool off in. We come in for a few hours' break and then we go back out in the evening. While playing on the playground, I also have her take rest breaks. A solid 40 minutes of climbing and running is plenty before she is zapped of energy. Again, we come back to the house and rest.

Since colds and flu are also a trigger for my daughter we choose to do a lot of our activities in the summer months when colds and flus are less frequent. We choose trips to the zoo, where we are surrounded by fresh air. I purposely choose to avoid crowded areas during cold and flu season and take full advantage of the spring and summer months.

Another thing I learned is that although I would like to celebrate holidays on the actual day itself, it is still just as much fun celebrating it on any day of the week. Children are happy if you are happy. They do not care what day you celebrate it so long as you acknowledge it. Many CVS kids end up spending holidays in the hospital due to excitement triggers. I do not even know the last time my daughter had a party on her exact birthday. The day we pick, however, is still just as much fun for her. Life can be just as fulfilling for a child with CVS.

Madeline: A Humorous Path
Paula Moss Dramm

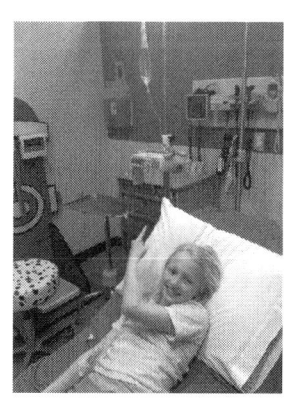

IV bag was better than finding an Easter basket.

We have spent many Christmas Eves, New Year's Eves, Valentines, family weddings and birthdays in an episode, but never Easter. We have traveled to my sister's house (two hour car ride from home) numerous times in my daughter's lifetime. But this time it was to celebrate a holiday and to see some of her favorite cousins that she hadn't seen in a while. It was a great time on Saturday night, playing board games with family and having many laughs. Madeline and her little five-year-old sister hardly remembered to even put out their Easter baskets for the Easter Bunny before going off to bed. The three of us dug our pajamas out of suitcases and went into the guest bedroom we were sharing. At 3:00 a.m. Madeline woke me up to say, "Mommy, I don't feel good." It was with that nervous-labored-breathing, almost-on-the-brink-of-tears voice, that voice CVS parents know all too well; and we knew it meant she was starting an episode.

I rushed to my box of abort medications that I thankfully remembered to pack. We tried it all, but she still threw up, luckily making it to the toilet because for the first time ever we were not at home for an episode. I was out of my element. I still had her throw up bucket in the car. My husband was two hours away because he had to work on Easter Sunday. We eventually moved to a family room in my sister's house and two more times she threw up that night, one time causing me to scrub my sister's bathroom floor and walls and use her washing machine. That feeling of not wanting to wake anyone else in the house up and yet wishing somebody else was up with you makes for a long night. Her little sister got up around 8:00 a.m., unphased that her sister was sick again, and proceeded to look for her Easter basket. But Madeline could care less where her basket even was. She was in pain and it hurt just to move. By 9:00 a.m. she threw up again, and I knew that I wanted to try to salvage this holiday and spend time with family. We needed to get to an ER. It's sometimes a tough call. Do I wait until she is fully dehydrated so the ER staff doesn't think I'm crazy for bringing a child in for an IV? Will her home abort drugs start to work? Or will I be sitting here two hours from now wishing I would have just gone to the ER sooner? So on Easter morning, instead of heading to a church called St. Mary's, I was headed to the ER of St. Mary's Hospital.

I had specific paperwork explaining what the ER doctor is supposed to give her along with labs that need to be done during an episode. But I forgot the papers at home. Luckily my husband was able to scan the papers in and email them to me before he went to work. Madeline could hardly walk into the ER. She was buckled over in pain and I was trying to support her and carry her throw up bucket in front of her mouth. She may have even looked like a kid that ate too much Easter candy. I was nervous. We were hours from home, we had never been to this ER, and all I had were photocopied orders from Madeline's CVS specialist.

Will the ER staff even know what CVS is and will they take my home printed copies of what medications to give seriously? Thankfully they did. They were a wonderful staff and said everything a CVS parent wants to hear. "Yes we have heard of it, but you probably know more about it than we do. You shouldn't have to convince us how to treat her. This paperwork is very helpful. You did the right thing. We will do all we can to get her feeling better fast." And they did. It was one of the fastest ER visits we ever had. I'm sure all the abort drugs I had given her at home helped the severity of the episode, but she still needed the fluids and the medication to go in her via IV or she would not have recovered that quickly. When a nine-year-old says "Can we go to the ER and get an IV," you know she must feel pretty bad. Before long she was sitting upright and smiling again. We joked that instead of finding an Easter basket that morning her treat was finding an IV. She agreed and was all smiles as the fluids and meds made her feel better. Which is why we took an Easter photo in the ER.

We were back to my sisters by 12:30 p.m. and able to have a great holiday with family. She even eventually remembered to look for her Easter basket, but knew she couldn't eat any of the treats that day. Holidays and family force you to count your blessings. We were blessed that day with a great medical staff, medications and orders from Madeline's CVS specialist that helped state our case and a quick recovery. We survived our first Easter episode and our first episode away from home.

Hope's Question: How to Explain CVS to a Child

From a young age CVS children know something is different. They watch others around them get sick and wonder why they are unable to do as well as others around them. Some may ask why, while other just assume it's their fault. This is why it is very important to affirm to our children that it is not them. Melissa Knight's daughter, at the age of four, brought this question up to her: Why does she get sick and end up in the hospital while her younger sister did not? How and when you explain CVS to your child varies, depending on the child's age and other circumstances. Below you find simple ways to reassure them that CVS does not mean that they are weak or the cause of the problem.

It's usually helpful to use analogies or simple stories to explain what is happening to a child. One analogy you could use is that of getting lost. Their brain's messages are getting a little lost and need help. Another useful analogy likens the average stomach flu to a windy day and CVS to a hurricane. They both present with the same problem (excessive wind), but differ in the intensity. One just causes minor challenges and is over quickly, while the other might knock out the power and keep you inside until the storm is over or cause an evacuation and requires more interventions and help to get through. It's important for them to realize that CVS is different.

Others might use the analogy of a battery. CVS cycles happen when your child's battery is not able to keep a good charge and the system starts to malfunction. The best way to recharge the battery and rest the system is to sleep. That is why your child might need you to make sure they rest often, eat often, and drink often to prevent the battery from reaching the low level. Everyone's batteries are a little different, and knowing what works best for your child is important to keeping them healthy. Everyone is made differently, so follow the directions that your child's body is telling them and don't worry about what others' bodies are telling them.

Remember to teach them to hold their heads high. Our children are not weak, they are riding out a storm that no one around them understands or sees the depth of.

Dana's Path: Courage Does Not Always Roar.
Dana Anelmo Pencak from Peaceloveparenthood.wordpress.com

Sometimes courage is the quiet voice at the end of the day saying…
"I will try again tomorrow"
~Mary Anne Radmacher

Meow. That's about all the roar I have in me some days. Sure, being courageous means standing strong, hanging tough and showing steadfast faith during trying times, but being brave can also be hard when we feel like we're at wit's end and all hope is gone. Whether it's a tragedy in our family, a job loss, a health crisis, a marriage on the rocks…or any of the large, medium or small issues we face in this world, let's be honest…it is REALLY hard to be courageous a lot of the time!

We've all had one of those days, weeks, months, even years where we just can't seem to get it together. When one door closes another door doesn't open, in fact we get multiple slams in our face day after day. We long for the light at the end of the tunnel or the shooting star to kickstart our faith. But it never comes. And we wait. Patiently at first, then when we realize all hope might be lost, we crumble. It's at those times in our lives where we have nothing else to do but find that inner strength, that call for courage so we can face each waking moment.

I love this quote because it's a wonderful reminder for all of us but especially appropriate when talking to children. When my kids are struggling with something my advice is usually, "Keep your chin up, lean on God and stay strong. Be courageous!" But we all know how tough that is to do. If we as adults can't find our way most days how in the world do we expect our kids to do the same?

You know what? I don't think there is an answer. I really don't think it's possible to be that perfect parent who is encouraging and motivating and loving and kind all wrapped up into one absolutely insanely courageous individual, at least on a consistent basis. No, it's not physically possible. Unless you're super mom or dad and if so, congratulations, your award is in the mail.

I think next time my kids face a closed-door or barricade on the road, I think I'll pay better attention to their roar or whimper and just be the quiet voice whispering in their ear…

No worries honey, tomorrow will be a better day. Tomorrow you can be courageous. And if not, there's always the next day and the next and the next. And you know what? It's going to be ok because you are loved.

Family Life

■ ■ ■

When a child has a chronic medical condition, its impact can be felt by everyone around them. It affects moms, dads, brothers, sisters, friends, and extended family as well. Adjusting to living with CVS can be hard on everyone. Siblings get used to not having mom or dad around because of being in the hospital often with their brother or sister. Our experiences might seem crazy and unique…..but from reaching out to other parents living with CVS we found again and again, our experiences are the same.

> Cycling Vomiting Syndrome has presented our whole family with a big challenge. We have no choice but to do what we have to so we get through each episode. We have had to rely on family and friends to mind Tara at a moment's notice. People have learnt that we will be there if we can but we are likely to cancel on them without any notice because Leonie is sick. We have learnt to make fun of the worst of situations.

> One of my best Mother's Days was getting breakfast in bed in hospital while Leonie was hooked up to a drip. Wayne brought Tara in to the hospital to visit and the four of us sat in Leonie's room and had dinner together. I didn't have to cook or clean all day. I have had the same treatment with at least one of my birthdays as have all family members. Our lives are full of frustration and disappointment but at the same time it has given our family a closeness that not all families have. We make the most of the well times and deal with

the sick times. It is no good complaining and there is always someone worse off than us.

—Anne Van Vilet

Blessings of Being a CVS Mom
Melissa Knight

I am a mother to two beautiful daughters. One of my daughters is diagnosed with CVS. Although I prefer to never hear the words cyclic vomiting, there are blessings that come from being introduced to it. Having a child with chronic medical conditions is exhausting, challenging, and at the same time, very rewarding. Looking back at my daughter's infancy, I have many memories that are filled with images of medical testing, procedures involving anesthesia, hospitalizations, and unknown worry.

Receiving a diagnosis of Cyclic Vomiting was difficult due to the vast amount of gastrointestinal issues she was experiencing on top of CVS. Nevertheless, after being able to put a name to the aggressive symptoms my little girl was experiencing, I became empowered with knowledge. It is always easier, once you attach a name to an illness, because at that very moment, the power shifts into your favor. You have the ability to research and seek out professionals and treatment options.

CVS has taught me to be present. Never do I take for granted watching my children play carefree in the backyard. I always smile seeing them singing their favorite songs, and tears are brought to my eyes after having a successful trip anywhere. I am thrilled to drive over a half hour without having to pull over due to my little one getting an abdominal migraine. I appreciate life every single day. I do so because the day could change as fast as a light switch. It can start off being fun and peaceful and end with a hospital admission. I live in the moment with each and every place we go. I experience the joy my children have and I feel it deep within my heart. I experience life as my children do and I mostly have pleasant memories in my mind now of happy times.

Having a child with CVS or any chronic medical condition can consume your life if you let it. It is important to research and become informed on CVS and it is equally important to adapt your life to allow your children to experience all of the joys life offers. A child who has CVS can still live a happy life.

Reflections of a CVS Mom
Jenny Granstrom

Ellie's health has been mediocre the last few weeks since the stomach flu/ER week. She has had a host of what I call "mini-episodes" where she gets very pale, very quiet, often has a low-grade fever and eventually gets teary and asks for her medicine, has to lay down with one of us, and all of us pray it passes. But more significant than the mini-episodes, she has had two more major episodes in the last month. A mini-episode is over in a few hours, but a major episode takes us down for 2-3 days, sometimes more depending on what the trigger is, like a virus for example. It also screws up our schedules and does a number on our sleep. So to experience a major episode every other week is a lot. My mommy definition of "more major" equates to total heartbreak with a side of puke and a LOT of stomach pain. Here are a few reflections on that:

1. The hard part about your child having a chronic illness is that it is chronic. I can't take it all away from her. When it's done it's not over. When we finish an episode we can't be comforted by thinking it won't happen again for a long, long time. Ellie recently shared with me (and her cute first grade class) that the worst part of living with CVS for her is always being worried that an episode might start: "Everyday I'm worried about it actually. I can't stop worrying about it."

So I remind her of how much we love her. I remind her again and again that she is so brave and so strong and that Daddy and I are so proud of her. I remind her that we will always stay with her. I remind her when we are chatting on a good day and I remind her when she is in the middle of it: "I'm here, honey, mommy's here. I'm so sorry. I know baby, I know. I'm right here."

And we brainstorm. I remind her that her teacher knows all about CVS and she can call me in an instant and that I will constantly check my phone in case her school calls. I write to her gym teachers to let them know she is having a hard time in gym lately. I ask them (beg, hope, pray) if they wouldn't mind reassuring her that it's ok for her to sit down, to get water, take a break. When going to playdates or birthday parties, I write down some info and my phone number and we tuck it in her pocket, just in case. Each morning I tell her to have a great day and then remind her that I'll be here if she needs anything. What more can we do? Recently I ordered a medical alert bracelet. It will be engraved with her health info and my phone number, I hope it brings her comfort.

2. Humans are naturally selfish, including me. When I write this blog, when I update friends and family, when I talk to the school nurse, I am always talking from my perspective. I say "it's hard" and "I'm exhausted," but in reality, I'm not in a massive amount of physical pain. I'm not the 7-year-old telling her class that she can't stop worrying about "it." I'm not walking around nauseous and tired with off and on stomach pain each day. How does she do it? If I puke once a year that is more than enough for me! Why am I complaining?

So I remind myself: I need to vent. For my whole life the very best way for me to move forward, to recharge and to stay strong has been for me to talk it out or write it out. This is how I remain strong so I can be strong when she needs me. I remind myself that it's ok that I am tired and it's ok that this is hard. I try to tell myself whatever it is that I would tell a friend who was going through the same thing: just because I am admitting that this is hard for me doesn't mean that I don't realize how much harder it is for her.

3. Just like Ellie, lately I feel like I have PTSD (post traumatic stress disorder). Ellie's episodes are trigger related, not over the same amount of days like some kids (in the CVS world, Ellie is a trigger-kid, not a calendar-kid), so I can't stop thinking about her triggers. It's always been on my mind to some degree since she was diagnosed, but the last few weeks, the chronic-ness of it all, my mind is a whirlwind. I can't stop wondering when another episode will start. I wonder how she is doing at school, I wonder whether she should do anything after school because of her poor energy lately, I wonder if it will be a bad night of sleep or a good one, I wonder if she is drinking enough, I wonder if she is being brave enough to ask to sit down during gym or dance class. I wonder if I should be calling the Milwaukee clinic to ask this question or that. When she looks tired, hot, or thirsty I immediately wonder if this is normal kid stuff or CVS-related and whether or not it will turn into anything.

Sooooo... I remind myself that she is strong. I remind myself that she is getting better and better at reading her own signals. I remind myself that we are doing our very best and that the most important thing is that she experience life to the fullest. CVS parents sometimes say that this disease can rob kids of their childhood. So we will control those triggers the best we can and then let her go ahead and run and play all the while crossing our fingers that things don't break bad in the middle of the night. I also remind myself that I need extra breaks; I need to laugh with my friends and think about other things.

While I can't take all this away from Ellie, I'm going to do everything in my power to make it better. I don't think this makes me unique. What loving parent doesn't want to make it better? But I do think I have been introduced to an intensity of that fix-it feeling that I would have been ok with skipping as far as parenting goes. I have this strong desire to think of new ways of making her more comfortable: different medicines, medical bracelets, cooling vests, e-mailing teachers, role playing with her how she might tell a teacher that she needs to sit down, etc, etc.

This year our family has also been working to raise money for the annual CVS run/walk. I made fliers to hand out to all the first-grade families at her school and she labeled envelopes to attach to the fliers. Then she and I gave a little presentation to her class about CVS. This had positive repercussions that I hadn't considered. For example, I was explaining to Ellie about a "cooling vest" (a little vest to wear on hot days or during hot activities. Cooling packs slide into pockets on the vest and it helps keep her body temperature down) and she said, "Well since everyone knows about my CVS now I think that is a really great idea. Now they know it's just what I have, right Mom?!" I was surprised; it hadn't occurred to me that she would be relieved that everyone knew about her CVS. I had been worried that she wasn't going to like the extra attention drawn to it. My Eleanor is strong, smart and brave.

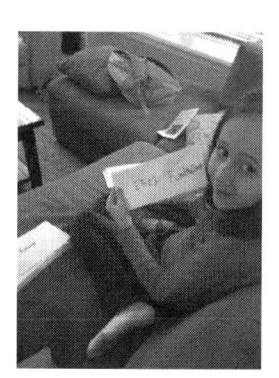

Motivated and excited.

Lastly, there is a sort of beauty to our interconnectedness, Ellie and I. On this Mother's Day weekend I would even say there is something transcendent, spiritual or otherworldly about it. I guess maybe it's cliché, but the longer I am a mom the more I understand that the love and connection between a mother and child cannot be compared to any other. No one can read Eleanor the way I can (My husband Brian is a close second of course). I am the first to recognize when she is a little "off" and I have recognized episodes that were hours away from starting. She has 10,000 facial expressions and I can probably interpret 9,500 of them. I can usually recognize the difference between a normal sequence of sleeping grunts and groans and a painful sequence of sleeping grunts and groans. And when I hold her hair back while she vomits, speak softly to her and sit by her bed for hours when she is moaning and crying through the night, there is a fire that lights between us. We are connected in a way that is hard to put into words.

I would pay all sorts of money, go through all sorts of hard labor, move away from all my family and friends, I would do pretty much anything to take this away from Ellie. That sounds dramatic but in the middle of a horrible episode it's the truth; however, I am grateful that this disease has forced me to recognize the fire-y connection between my children and myself. They are my everything, an extension of my heart.

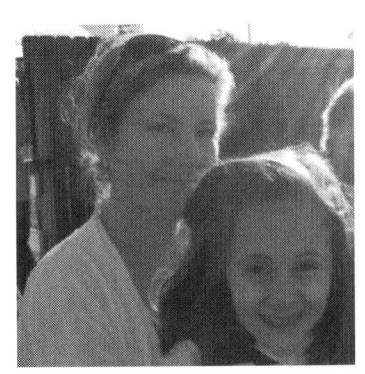

Rice Family New Additions

From May to June of 2013, was an exciting time in the Rice household. In early May we welcomed a new member, Julianne. Throughout my whole pregnancy I worried, what if I were to go into labor while I was caring for Andrew in the hospital. What did happen was something I

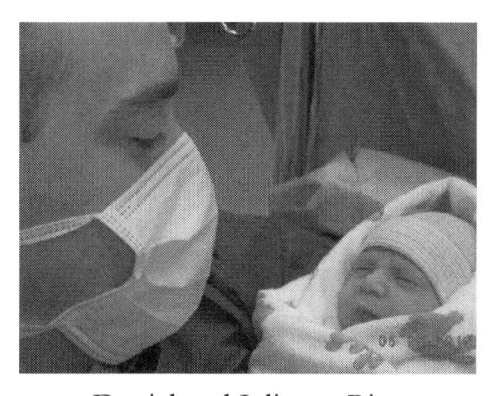

Daniel and Julianne Rice

had not even considered. My husband I arrived at the hospital early in preparation for my scheduled c-section. We were relieved that Andrew had not gotten sick during the night, we thought maybe, just maybe, CVS would skip us this time. Everything with the surgery had gone well and Julianne was doing well. Dan left around 11 to go to Andrew's school to pick him up to bring him to meet his newest sister. Andrew had worked very hard to earn this prize and was the first to hold her. When he came in he was excited, happy, but very pale. He smiled as he held her and helped daddy change her diaper. He then skipped out happily as he left. I wanted to breathe a sigh of relief, but something was still off about him. As soon as he got home, he fell asleep from all the excitement (which is our first sign of an impending cycle). The CVS had hit after the delivery.

    The vast majority of the time I had been Andrew's advocate, only because I knew the doctors there very well. This time I would have to let go and allow daddy to advocate for him. Dan was more than capable of doing it. My mom was home with our other four children, while Julianne and I were in the maternity wing, and Dan was with Andrew in the emergency room. I had to trust and let go of what little control I had gotten used to having. Sometimes the staff were those who knew Andrew and his history, and other times not. If you are the primary caregiver you understand how hard it was for me. All I could do was have them call me if they had any questions since I physically could not go down to the emergency room. I had made sure to lay out his treatment plan and folder earlier that morning, but in all the excitement it was left at home.

Andrew, Julie, and I remained in the hospital recovering for the next 4 days. Happily we were all discharged the same day. However the next few weeks, we would make frequent trips to the hospital with a 1-2 day stay each time. The nurses, thankfully, were wonderful, and would put a newborn open crib in the room for Julie to sleep in while we were there. We had developed a healthy sense of humor and rolled with it during that time. I think back now and wonder how we ever managed all that. Somehow we did. Being a mom can have its challenging moments. At those times, I am so thankful I have a supportive husband, and my own mother who is able to jump in and lend a hand.

Natalie's Path: A Father's Perspective
Mike Dion

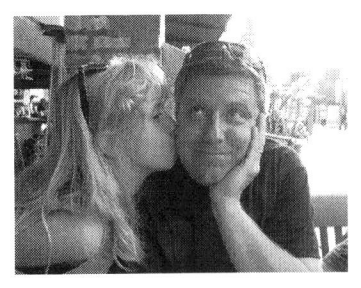

My daughter Natalie is nine and a half. She started screaming and was full of life from the moment she was born, and from that very moment I knew that my wife and I were going to be in for a long haul. At the time, these imagined challenges were concerns about boys, teenage attitude, and difficulty with friends.

Although she has always had random medical issues, her current illness started during a run on Thanksgiving Day almost three years ago. Natalie started throwing up and did not stop for the entire weekend. As an RN, I saw this as one of the many issues that happen during childhood. Kids get the flu, gastroenteritis, and a host of other things from other kids. That weekend we took her to the emergency room to stop the throwing up. We were told that Natalie did in fact have one of those childhood illnesses. She had strep throat. I thought, great, bring on the antibiotics, and let's get on with the weekend. We were released to go home. When we arrived home Natalie started throwing up again. I felt like a failure as a nurse because all the things I knew to do when a kid is sick were not working. Eventually we had to take her back to the hospital, this time to be admitted.

To avoid being long winded, the next six months involved many different doctors with each one wanting a new test. Along the way, Natalie's nausea never left. Around every Wednesday, Natalie would be extremely tired and sometimes take a three hour nap. When she woke up, she would still be tired and still have the nausea. After many tests and many instances of finally "finding a cause and a cure," our hopes were let down with continued nausea, constant fatigue, and a litany of doctors shaking their heads, and saying they just did not know.

By the time we checked our daughter for cancer, specifically leukemia, I almost hoped it would be cancer so we would have an answer, and a possible cure. It was about this time that my daughter's confidence, lust for life and "I can do anything" attitude started to leave. In the place of a bold, precocious child, we had a sensitive, scared, anxiety-ridden little girl. Natalie worries about everything. She has a nervous habit that causes her to pick her skin, and when it scabs, she picks it again. Many times, she has no idea she is doing it; when you tell her to stop, she looks at her fingers, ashamed. This was the worst thing to see. There is a very real stigma in society regarding psychiatric conditions. I did not want that for my daughter.

When we saw new doctors this new anxiety was part of the health history. Unfortunately, this caused some of the more "shortsighted" doctors to write off the nausea, extreme fatigue, severe vomiting as anxiety. This is garbage. My kid did not develop anxiety and nervousness until being told for six months that we were no closer to finding out what was wrong.

It did not help that I did not understand the irrational fears and anxiety either. I would get angry at Natalie, she would start to cry and say that I "just don't understand, don't you realize dad, I hate this nausea. I hate being this way." Natalie wanted to know why God was doing this to her. I had no real answer. No answer except for the usual crappy response, "one day God will let us know." I used to feel that God was a kid with a magnifying glass on an anthill. I started to think that way again. Some days, my child could not even ride in the car for fear of throwing up in the car. I just wanted my kid back. Natalie just wanted to be a kid again. The things she used to do like sleepovers, school, sports, even movies with friends did not happen anymore. If she did anything, mom had to be close by.

We saw a pediatric neurologist who asked questions but did not wait for the answers. When he did hear the answers, he dismissed them. He put Natalie on Topamax, a seizure medication that took away the nausea, but turned Natalie into a zombie. She went from being an "A" student to a "C" student. Problem solving was non-existent. Natalie's teachers said that she looked "zoned out" in class. We looked up the side effects of this medication when she started taking it. We knew this was a risk, but at higher doses. When we asked the neurologist about this, he dismissed the possibility outright while at the same time telling us that the "blunted" way Natalie was behaving was the new normal! We were not ok with this "new normal," which was obviously caused by medicine side effects.

Eventually we found a doctor that was able to confirm a diagnosis for us. Natalie had Cyclic Vomiting Syndrome, a mitochondrial disorder. The mitochondrion is the powerhouse of the cell. This is the reason we are able to do anything at all. The specialist, Dr. Boles, put Natalie on a "mito cocktail" that really helped. The nausea never left, but was very well managed. In addition he took Natalie off the Topamax. He referred to this drug as "stupidmax." Guess what? The "new normal" as described before went away. The old Natalie started to come back. Confidence returned, Natalie's fears subsided, and I felt we had an answer. We were so glad to have our daughter back.

Then last May, 2012, Natalie got way worse. Everything described above returned, but much, much worse. Natalie's specialist explained that this was due to the rise in hormones and was in fact truly, "the new normal." During the summer Natalie stayed in the hospital for nine days. We were back to where we were before we had Natalie on the mito cocktail. Everything that worked for a year and a half before was no longer working. New issues came up, many of them including dysautonomia, a dysfunction of the autonomic nervous system. For the first time, Natalie got her typical nausea with an addition of a severe headache. Now the headaches did not go away either. Natalie asked me if she was going to die. I said no. What else do you say? Sometimes, it's OK to lie to your kids. The truth is that I have no idea where this is going.

One of the hardest parts of this illness was the insurance company. They told us they would not cover the expense to see Dr. Boles. This is the one doctor that kept Natalie OUT of the hospital for over a year!!! If anything, we saved them money by decreased visits to the ED for fluids and medications with eventual admissions to the hospital. This was despite the fact that every specialist the insurance company wanted us to see was telling us to see Dr. Boles!! Yet still the battle continued.

I have some sadness in me these days. My daughter has been cheated out of a normal life. I even prayed to God to heal Natalie and give the illness to me. He did not hear me. I sort of thought that if you selflessly asked for something, you could get it. I have a child-like faith. Only a child would believe such a thing. My son suffers because my daughter's issues consume our lives. We are getting better about making plenty of time for him. My marriage suffers because my daughter's issues consume our lives. I could not tell you the last time my wife and I have had a date. It would be cool if the damn insurance company would just approve her specialist. My daughter may never be able to be on her own. This has changed her life. It has changed our lives.

The point of writing this is not for sympathy. It is to say to other families dealing with chronic illness that I sort of get their lives now. I am slowly learning to appreciate where I am because it could absolutely get worse. Something is happening to our kids in this country. Autism, Mitochondrial disorders, ADHD, ADD. I sense something is affecting the genetic makeup of our children. I could not tell you if it is the water, genetically altered food, chemicals, pesticides, or all of these. I wish we knew so we could do something about it.

My daughter was watching the "fab five" show – the USA Gymnastics team who had won gold in the Olympics. My daughter loved gymnastics, but was now too completely fatigued to take part anymore. Natalie was afraid to go that night. She started crying, and did not want to get sick at the performance. Her mom and I made her go. Don't give in to the fear. "Dad, will I be ok?" "Yeah, you be will fine," I answer back. Sometimes it's OK to lie to your kids.

A Grandmother's Point of View
Jack's Grandma

Even to this day, I remember the excitement, pride and love I felt the day my daughter gave birth to her first child. This is a blessing all mothers look forward to. Overwhelmed with joy, I held that little bundle in my arms with a grateful prayer in my heart for this new life.

From about the time Jack turned a year old, I had a hint that something was wrong. My daughter often mentioned Jack getting sick during the night. After repeated times of telling me this, I told her I didn't think this was normal and she attributed it to Jack being a day-care baby and that he was picking up the "bug" there.

This "bug" continued to recur much too frequently and I began to notice, at times, a strange gaze in Jack's eyes. Often he would not respond to his name. Autism? As I look back now and think about the first years of his life, it's difficult to remember all the quirks in his behavior that one would generally not see in a toddler.

The circumstances around Jack's illness are likely similar to other children who suffer from CVS. To write about it in more detail would only confirm the same story others have to tell. Instead, I'd like to approach this writing by telling you what I've experienced happening to my daughter, Jack's mother.

There isn't a day when she isn't advocating for her son. From the time he was approaching the end of his first year of life and his CVS symptoms appeared, she reached out to every doctor, resource, and website for information and help. One doctor after another seemed to be dumbfounded and couldn't provide any explanation or solution. From pediatricians, neurologists, gastrologists, hearing specialist, and many others, each had an opinion but none provided an answer. What we've learned in the meantime is that most doctors don't have the background necessary nor were they willing to admit their lack of knowledge regarding Cyclic Vomiting Syndrome.

My daughter works in a health care profession and she was personally witnessing the fact that an answer isn't always easy to come by. The months and years passed and doctor after doctor couldn't seem to pinpoint a diagnosis. How the help finally came isn't important here. What is important is that she persisted and persisted and persisted until "bingo."

When you have a sick child or one that seems to have unusual medical issues, the obvious answer in getting help is to see a doctor. I am sure all the other moms of children suffering from CVS find themselves in the same situation as my daughter. Who knows about this disease until you've researched and researched?

The child suffers from CVS, but so do his mommy and daddy. It is not easy to watch repeatedly, month after month after month, these episodes. I've only witnessed three but I can say they are unbearable to watch. Your heart breaks again and again. Of course, the child needs to be cared for, but so do his parents. My support and assistance are often long distance because of where I live and, for that reason, I too feel helpless.

Always, when I tell my friends, neighbors and others about Jack's illness, they say, "Cyclic Vomiting Syndrome, never heard of it. What's that?" When will that change? So much time and suffering for both patient and parents could have been avoided if only (why are there always so many "if onlys" in life) that first doctor had been familiar with CVS.

Taylors Grandma: Poetic Path
Rhonda Feasel, Ohio USA

Puke Monster, Puke Monster

Please go away,
For I just wanna
Be normal for a day.
I didn't invite you
To enter my life,
I didn't ask for all
Your strife.
I don't know why you
Have to be so mean,
I don't understand
Why you chose me.
I want you to leave
Because today,
I want to be a kid
And run and play.
But here I am
Sick once more,
I wish you would leave
Straight out the door.
Never to return
For I don't want you here,
I'm tired of being sick
And my family living in fear.
So Puke Monster, Puke Monster
Please go away,
Because I wanna be normal
Just for a day.

Cyclic Vomiting and Extended Family

When a child is sick it affects more than just the child. It affects the caregivers, parents, siblings, grandparents and close friends. Often when a child is sick with a chronic condition such as CVS, families become afraid to make plans for fear of another "episode" ruining events. Since many children take their emotional cues from those around them, it is important to realize what impact those around us have on how well our children deal with chronic medical conditions.

Melissa Knight shares how those around her did "not understand why we miss out on family activities and parties and the seriousness of what a simple runny nose could do to our daughter." We should try to surround ourselves with as many people who "get it" as we can. This may mean distancing ourselves from others who may think we are making our child sick, or that we are using CVS as an excuse to get out of attending an event or family gathering. This could be a huge help in conserving our emotional and physical energy since we are already maxed out at is it.

Sometimes family members can be a blessing when they offer to help out by cooking a meal or taking a sibling to school or practice. They also can be a source of stress when they make harsh judgments about us as parents, citing us as the problem and poor parenting as the reason our children are sick. Worse yet, they sometimes say we are taking our child to the hospital in an effort to gain attention. They have not seen our child during episodes and choose not to come around.

In my family my dad did not acknowledge CVS as real medical condition until my son was diagnosed doing the same thing I had done as a child. He held on to the notion that I was just a stubborn child and that what my son had was different. Eventually I think he came around, and just loved to tease me about it. I don't think he understood at the time how much the validation meant to me. I don't think he started to get it until I started writing this book. Not until I shared with him my conversations with parents from other countries did he see it as something that really was real. He's coming around now, which might be later than I would have liked, but I'm still relieved.

Ways Others Can Support Us

One day I came across an article *Dear People Who Do Not Have a Child with Disabilities* on the blog nopointsforstyle.com. In her blog, Adrienne writes about things she's learned from raising her child who has health and developmental challenges. Her child does not have CVS, but many of her points are helpful. We have probably all wished the people around us better understood these unique challenges we are going through as parents of child with disabilities or health concerns. Often those around us don't know what say to us when we share that our child is sick again. Adrienne's post gives us some specific things we could mention to others as ways to support and encourage us.

- Listen. Just listen. Open yourself up. Yes, it hurts and it's very scary. That's OK. There is a person in front of you who is in pain. Don't leave her alone with it.
- Know that you can't fix it. Don't try. We have doctors and therapists and other professionals for treatment. Also, that diet/book/supplement you heard about that can cure all the problems? We've heard of it already. We're on the internet while you sleep, and anyway, 26 of our Facebook friends already sent us the link.
- Acknowledge and affirm. Say, *wow, that sounds hard*. Say, *oh, my God, how painful!* Say, *I hate that it's so difficult for you*.
- Treat our kids the same way you treat other children in your life. Of course you should be sensitive, especially with kids who have emotional/social/behavioral issues, because many of them don't want to be touched or may not be verbal, but in general, if you usually engage kids in conversation, do that with our

kids too. Say hello. Smile. They might not respond predictably, if they respond at all, but they see you.

- Offer to help, but only if you mean it (people in pain are sensitive; we know when you're saying words you don't mean so you can feel good about yourself). My mom sometimes came to my house and gathered all my laundry baskets and every scrap of dirty laundry in the house (which completely filled the trunk of her car) and brought it all back a day or two later, clean and folded. As much as I appreciated the clean clothes, meals, and rides, I was even more grateful to feel a little less alone in the world.

- Send a note, a text, or an email. Parenting a child with special needs can be profoundly lonely. It's also hectic and chaotic and we may not respond to you, but do it anyway. The world starts to feel very far away when life is all appointments, crisis, chaos, and praying for survival. Stay connected, even if it feels one-sided.

- If you're very close, spend a little time learning about your friend's child's diagnosis. There is no need to become an expert, but an evening spent learning will only make you a better listener. If you don't know what to read, your friend will gladly tell you.

- Keep listening. Just show up and listen. There's nothing any person in pain needs more.

Top 10 Ways We Can Explain and Educate Others about CVS

As a parent of a CVS child we get lots of advice and suggestions from doctors, nurses, friends, teachers, and family. Some recommendations are helpful, others are not. Having a child with a chronic condition can wear you down physically and emotionally and can make you want to scream when encountering others who don't "get it." Here's a list of the top 10 misunderstood things about CVS and suggestions on how to respond:

1. *It's "just" a stomach virus.*

    While viruses can be a trigger, vomit related to CVS does not look or smell the same. CVS children puke up to 20x an hour, not a day, and they dehydrate much faster than non-CVS children. CVS is not just a stomach virus, and it's not repeated food poisoning and in most cases not a food allergy either.

2. *Oh, I can relate. My kid had a stomach flu once and we missed a special birthday party.*

    Many CVS kids spend holidays admitted to the hospital, hooked up to an IV, and sedated. They're not at home with family. They *regularly* miss graduations, First Communions, first days of school, birthday parties, vacations, field trips, summer camps, etc. It's not that we mean to be insensitive...or even that you mean to. We would LOVE to be able to have a child who was occasionally mildly sick and sometimes we get frustrated. Forgive me if I snap at you.... or need to bite my tongue.

3. *Has your child ever had an IV before or been in the Emergency Room?*

    Many well intentioned nurses have asked us this. The answer to most CVS kids will be a YES. To even have CVS on a chart means we have gone months or years of being dismissed as merely having a stomach virus, flu etc. and have been treated or seen in the ER more than most.. So, yes, you can rest assured the child has had an IV before...Our CVS friend Sean has been known to tell the nurses what size or gauge of needle works best for him and which veins are most cooperative.

4. *Do not tell us "they grow out of it" or quote studies that many kids do and then do nothing to help us when we are having a cycle.*

This may be true, but for now CVS is wreaking havoc on our lives. Right now we need help making a plan to manage this. We have simple goals, like to make it six weeks without a cycle or hospital admission. We want to get through a holiday or birthday just once. We're not really that focused on the "someday" or "by teen years." Someday sounds nice, but we'd like a nice week or month without it now. We rejoice in simple things, such as when we are able to abort an episode at home or are only admitted two days instead of four. We long for that day when this will be a distant memory, but the day we're in the ER is obviously not this day. Please help us get through today.

5. *I did not call you because I know you're used to it by now.*

   We may have the hospital routine down to a fine art. We do still like to be validated by a phone call, text, or email. We love to have a meal dropped off at home or at the hospital for us. As used to it as we become, it's still exhausting and lonely as we sit in our quiet dark hospital rooms for days at a time.

6. *It's all in your kid's head or it's an anxiety thing that you are causing.*

   Well, yes, stress is a trigger, but it is not the main cause for CVS. Everyone gets stressed but not everyone retches blood and vomits 10x an hour for days if not treated. Stress aggravates the condition and can make it more difficult to manage, but it's not the cause itself. True, in early days, we make a lot of mistakes, but GOD WILLING we learn what we can do to minimize. Some of us learn quicker than others. Encourage us to do what we need to do. This might mean homeschooling, being homebound, or other things you might consider different from the norm.

7. *The kids would be fine if you just gave them sips of water every five minutes.*

   This is good in theory for the regular stomach flu, but not so for CVS kids. For us and many others, even small sips trigger retching, aggravating the vomiting cycle process. This is why we go into the hospitals to prevent dehydration, kidney failure, and other complications. If the kids could drink, they surely would. During a cycle, CVS kids often crave fluids and would do anything to have the mere ability to drink and have it stay down. (Congratulations to those who are able to take sips).

8. *He or she is only being stubborn—Swallow your saliva kid!*

The inability to swallow is not a sign of stubbornness or defiance when it comes to CVS. It's actually something that most of us take for granted and do without thinking. For CVS kids, swallowing becomes not so automatic for them after hours of painful retching. Hyper-salivation is a telltale sign of CVS, making the problem worse. Swallowing is a mind-over-matter thing at some level, but it's a lot more than that...and it's far from being a problem of stubbornness (though on other matters I'm sure many of these kids are very stubborn).

9. *They are just vomiting to get attention because of X Y Z.*

Emotional changes that come along with having a new brother or sister, a move, a divorce or death in the family, or new teacher at school trigger cycles. It is not that children want more attention. They just want to feel better and eat, drink and play like everyone else.

10. *You need to find a better doctor.*

CVS is a chronic condition without a cure. There is no simple answer to the problem of CVS as of yet. There is no DOCTOR who has the perfect cure for every single child with any illness. Our medical teams work very hard for us and with us to help minimize its impact. However, life is life. It's exciting and full of things that set CVS off. Some days you win, some days you don't. It's not our doctor's fault, or even ours...we are all doing everything we can to reduce the impact of CVS. Sometimes it's just matter of time and documenting how each of the meds work.

The Sibling Experience

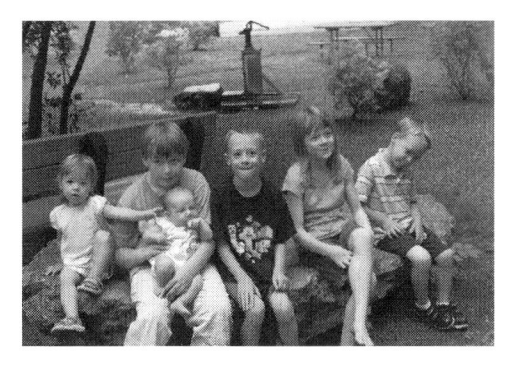

In our large family of six kids, it's a quite the juggling act when Andrew is in the hospital. Thank God for grandparents who live close by and are able to step in whenever needed. It has also been interesting watching how the other kids respond to seeing Andrew so sick. They have been known to run for the towels or to help pack a bag quickly. They also have learned to spot their brother's warning signs.

They are all learning compassion and how to care for the sick. When he is well, Andrew is the first to offer assistance to his other siblings if they are sick. Yes, there are missed events that occur, as well as some hurt feelings from time to time. We are fortunate to have a supportive family and usually find a way to make sure each kid gets what they need. Also remember CVS changes with time so we take full advantage of the good times when we can.

Our youngest daughter, Julianne, probably spent more time in the hospital than at home during her first month of life. I would bring a pack and play and set it up in the room. She was breast feeding so leaving her home was not an option. Since Andrew loved her, it was a good thing to motivate him to do what he needed to get better so that he could play with her again. That worked for about the first 8 months of her life... then she got chatty and things got challenging again.

I was glad to connect with Anne Van Vilet who actually

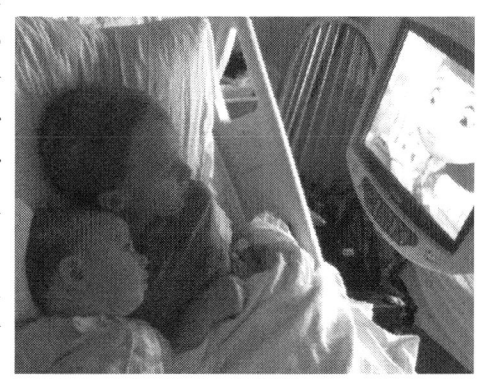

had gone through a similar experience with her daughters. She shared with me that:

> Leonie has a sister Tara who is almost 4 years younger than her. Tara has grown up knowing that if her sister wakes up vomiting she will most likely be in hospital that night. Tara was only two weeks old when Leonie had one of her episodes. As I would stay in the hospital with Leonie Tara stayed as well. The nursing staff wheeled in a cradle from the maternity ward and Tara slept in the room with us. After that I would express bottles and have them in the freezer so that her father Wayne and her grandparents could look after Tara while I managed Leonie. We would never have survived those times without the support of our extended family and friends. We would have a call list to phone around for people to have Tara come and stay with them while we dealt with getting Leonie well again

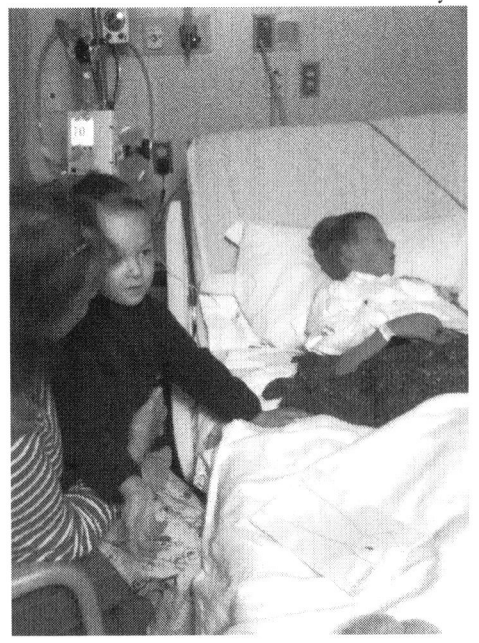

Newborns and toddlers might not remember or know anything different but life with a chronically ill sibling. The experience of siblings who are older is a different story. I sat down with my oldest son, to get his thought of what was going on with his brother. Matthew was about 8 when Andrew started have frequent cycles that required hospitalization. He mentioned that he was concerned that his brother was never going to come home after a weeklong hospital stay. Our daughter Kate, who is a year younger than Matthew, had a hard time understanding why Andrew did not go to school. She felt like he was missing out on the fun of school, and at other times, tried to fake being sick so she could homeschool as well. Gregory went to school in tears one day because he missed Andrew during a hospital admission. We had to break the no visitor rule we had created for him. Once he saw his brother and gave him a card he made for him, he felt much better.

After about six months of repeated admissions, our kids had become so familiar with it they no longer were shocked. They learned what CVS was and that taking Andrew to the hospital was the way to keep Andrew safe when he got sick. They did become worried, as they watched him continue to lose weight and get weaker and weaker. It was hard to reassure them he was going to be ok, when we were wondering the same thing.

But what is a parent to do? How are you supposed to juggle the needs of all your children? When you're sleep deprived and caring for your sick child consumes all of your energy, the last thing you want is to have to worry about your other children. Below are some tips that have helped us to make sure our other children's needs are being met.

1. Remember to ask for help. It's not possible to do it all when a child is sick. Don't feel bad about asking for help. You can ask extension on school projects for siblings if you are stuck in the hospital and not able to be home to help. Ask a friend to do carpool line

2. Try to take time to have one on one with your other children even if it's a phone call, a message or a special treat you leave for them. I used to bring home the baby coke cans from hospital trays or split special desserts with them if they did come to visit.

3. If your hospital has free Wifi or you have a smart phone, make use of the variety of video chat apps out there. Sometimes just connecting in this way can help a child feel better about the time you are away.

4. Remind them that they are loved just as much as the sick sibling. They would want you to be with them if they were the sick one.
5. Allow them to talk openly about how they feel even if its angry, sad, scared. If you are unable to talk to them about this, you can ask for help from school counselors or other adults that they trust and feel safe with. No matter how much they might say it does not bother them, know that it does.

A Cure For CVS

By Emily Bell
Age 14, 9th Grade, CVS Sibling

Today I can write lines of a tortured boy.
Write for example, our lives have exploded.
Hospital visits, doctors' appointments, and pain in control.
A pale miserable face confined to a dark silent room.
Today I can write lines of a tortured boy.
I weep for him and occasionally he weeps for me.
Through the months of pain and misery I try to console
those hopeless eyes.
If only my prayers could end his suffering.
He weeps for me and occasionally I weep for him.
How could God make him experience such excruciating pain?
Today I can write lines of a tortured boy.
Why must this happen to such an innocent soul?
If only my words and prayers could heal his pain
and return my brother to me.
Moaning and screaming in pain.
What can I do?
How could no one fix this evil disease?
Today I can write lines of a tortured boy.
His pain and misery spreads throughout the family.
No one can help.
Nothing we can do.
Cyclic Vomiting Syndrome you have caused
this pain in an innocent boy.
You EVIL disease!

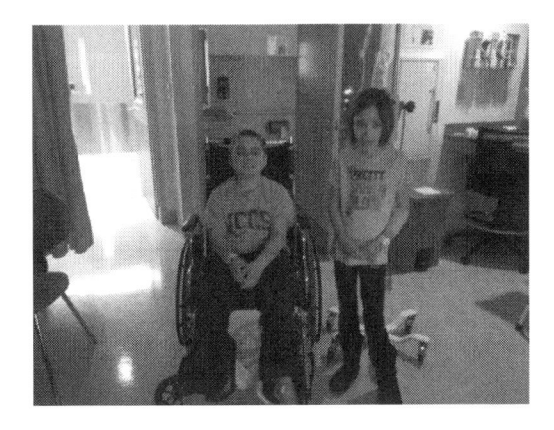

CVS sibling Adam and Lauryn Bell, Siblings of Emily Bell Double admission..... Poor parents but they lived through it!

The Education Question for CVS kids

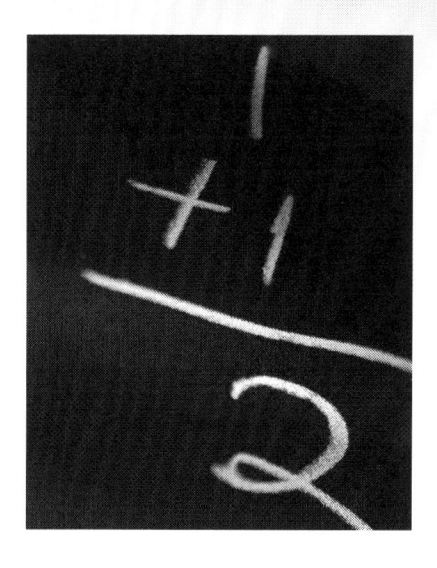

Kids do not remember what you teach them, but what you are.

Jim Henson

Dare to Think Differently

One blessing I think CVS and functional mitochondrial disorders have done for our family is that it has made us take brave steps to think differently than we otherwise would have done. Yes, we all can list the things we have not been able to do because CVS. Many of these children spend days hooked up to IVs, while their peers are out playing freely. This has an impact on them in so many ways. How can we as parents compensate for this somewhat lost or compromised childhood? Can we?

Because my son cycles frequently and requires many hospitalizations, we made the last minute decision to homeschool him this past September after attending his first grade open house. As expected, we got the 4:00 a.m. puke wakeup call and were in the emergency room by the time he should have been getting ready for his first day of first grade. This proved to be a six day hospital admission. I thought and thought as we struggled to get the puking under control in the hospital, and I knew something had to give. Something had to be different, outside of the box, otherwise I feared I'd just be moving into Southern New Hampshire Medical center for the school year because his cycles would surely increase.

But homeschooling? Could I really do it and take care of his five siblings? Well honestly, it could not possibly be worse than the track we were heading on if we stayed this course. Coming off of a horrible spring and summer, Andrew was in no way ready to start first grade, in which the focus would be on his weakest areas, handwriting and reading. First grade students are supposed to be able to write letters, and be willing to learn to read. Andrew was a young boy who learned hands on and who does not respond well to demands being placed on him unless he was able to do it perfectly. School, therefore, as it was being presented to us at this time, was MASSIVE TRIGGER that we would be dealing with every day.

We decided to focus on his health that year by taking what is known as a Grace Year, where he was allowed to explore topics of his choosing in the way he chose. We create scenes with the building blocks and then write stories about it together. We read classics like *Ralph S. Mouse*, *Trumpet of the Swan*, *Geronimo Stilton* books, and many more. He was assigned things to build on the popular Minecraft. It was a wonderful year of exploring things at the pace he set. He finally gained weight and was back up to a healthy BMI (body mass index). He still had frequent hospital stays, but the length of time he was sick decreased greatly. He was happy, and he was actually eating enough food to sustain him! He finally was able to have a more balanced energy level. Sure, he was only starting to sound out words, but he was in a better place and ready to learn now, where he would otherwise not have been. He came so far with the goals that we set for him, many of which people might take for granted, such as eating a meal, drinking enough when healthy, and just less frequent hospital stays.

This might sound like a no brainer but many of you know how challenging it can be get a CVS child to eat. For some it's because they cycle so rapidly, for others a fear of eating develops, and for still others there is ongoing pain that prevents them from getting what they need to get stronger. After two years crazy of frequent cycles and numerous hospital admissions, I've come to a huge realization. Andrew did not finally start to truly rebound until recently when for whatever reason he was finally able to begin to eat normally. Our break in the cycle came when we focused on getting back to normal rather than keeping up with where he "should be." We placed our focus on helping him become happy and healthy by the creative approach of a grace year, where we did more of a student-directed study. We reduced his stress by scaling back the demands that were placed on him and allowing him to set the pace. For us this worked wonderfully! I feel like now he is ready to move on to a different learning environment.

As a CVS parent you probably have struggled with trying to sort out what your child's triggers are and how to avoid them all while trying continue to lead the normal life we had before the CVS for the rest of family. Sometime this is near impossible and changes and accommodations need to be made, and that need not be considered a failure. Seeking alternatives for the time being was the best thing we could have done.

Leonie's School Path.
Anne Van Vliet

Leonie has missed a lot of school time. We are fortunate enough that we live in a rural town with a small primary school of about 200 students. We were not able to get funding for a teacher's aid but the principal would make sure that Leonie would be put in a class with an aid funded student so that she could get extra assistance to help her catch up after being away. We would always get work sent home and would get some private tutoring for her. The teachers would keep a close eye on Leonie and make sure that she was eating and drinking and call us if she was not feeling too well.

Knowing that Leonie would get lost in a large public secondary school with over 1200 students we chose a small independent Christian school for Leonie's secondary school. They have been very helpful and gone out of their way to help Leonie keep up with her school work. Now that she is getting to the serious end of her schooling it is getting harder to keep up with work missed from being away. Leonie emails her teachers and they send her work. I spend a lot of time helping with school work. I read each novel Leonie reads and we sit and discuss the books and throw ideas around together like they would in the class room. Her school also provides her some time with a tutor as well as dropping subjects that she does not really need to do. We have discussed a plan to help get her through year 11 next year and she will most likely do year 12 over two years to ease the work load and take off the pressure that goes with this year. Leonie does not know what she wants to do after that but at the moment she would like it to involve ballet.

We have let Leonie be involved in as much as she can at school. She has always gone on excursions and camps. I have gone along on a few of the camps with her but sometimes the schools have been happy to take her on her own if she has been well in the lead up to the camp. We often tell the story of having to drive three hours one night to go and pick Leonie up from a school camp after she had been vomiting all day. We were at the camp long enough to have a cup of coffee then drove the two and a half hours back to the hospital. That was a long trip back with a very sick child but at least the teachers now know what happens when she gets sick.

Brady's Path: The School Nurse Can't Handle This
Kandy Wesson

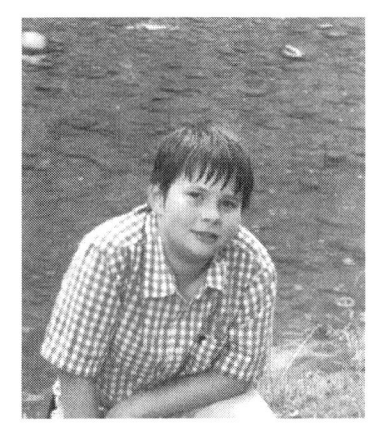

Brady entered this world five-and-a-half weeks early. I had pre-eclampsia, and he was born via C-section. He had his first endoscopy at two weeks old. The doctors told us it was just really bad reflux. As he grew, he was always in the bottom or even under the growth charts for his age. He "spit up" a lot. Sometimes, God would wake me to suction his poor mouth and nose out, or he wouldn't be here today. We heard the terms "colic" and "GERD" so many times it was unreal. I knew there was more, and that beyond the tummy issues, there were behavioral issues.

Brady got diagnosed with autism at three years old. I had to change his daycare when I changed jobs. I chose a cutesy daycare with little white picket fences to section off each room. There was even a floor to ceiling slide with ball-pit! What child would not just love this, right? Wrong, so wrong. He was happy at first. The second week I started receiving phone calls. Your baby is sick. You need to pick him up. No fever, just miserable, and spitting up. He had only been hospitalized a couple of times at this point.

Fast forward to when he was seven. Constant vomiting, crying all the time. Was it the autism? Was it a stomach virus? Was his immune system just too weak to fight off any virus he encountered? We get sent to a GI doctor. He diagnoses Brady with Celiac Disease. We went on a gluten-free diet. His symptoms seemed to improve some, but we still had several 3-5 day hospital stays. We maxed out missing about 30 days of school that year. You know, every time a kid vomits, it's a virus. I almost got fired from my job due to being "not dependable." I changed jobs, and happened to be placed at my son's school.

Wonderful! I am here! I can fix it! I can give him extra meds when he needs them. He can even come and sleep on the trampoline in the special ed room I work in, so he doesn't miss any more school.

Wrong again. Well, right that I gave him meds, and he didn't miss as much, but he was miserable! About 3-4 days a week, he came to my room to get "headache" medicine. I would give him some ibuprofen and send him on his way. At least three days a week, he returned to my room, with a bucket to vomit in by the trampoline. Yes, I got to work, but what was the purpose of him being at school? He slept most of the time, so he wasn't learning much.

Sadly, my husband and I separated and I moved across town. I decided to go ahead and transfer Brady while I worked at the other school, 45 minutes away. I had an IEP meeting with the staff at the school, and informed them of the protocol I used when he got sick. Anxiety is a huge trigger for him, and I warned them. Really, I did.

The first two weeks were wonderful! Only one phone call because he had an autism meltdown. I got him calmed down and hoped that would be the way the rest of the year would go. After two weeks, the monster struck more violently than ever before. The school called me. I wasn't close enough to give him abortive meds. I thought he had a "nervous stomach." He would vomit about 10 times before I could pick him up. Then, in the middle of March, the school nurse called and said, "I do not know how this little guy can produce so much vomit! He's vomited about 21 times in the past hour." She called me again while I was on my way to pick up to inform me that he was vomiting blood. We went straight to Children's Hospital.

We finally started receiving answers after his upper GI was performed for a third time at nine years old. No Celiac Disease! Wow! Ok, I'll take that! His esophageal sphincter was so weak, the doctor said if he wasn't nine years old, he would diagnose him as a bulimic. Then he mentioned possible CVS. What? The pharmacy?? I'm confused. The doctor then explained cyclic vomiting to me. Brady had lost about 12 lbs at this point. With some new preventative meds and new abortive meds for abdominal migraines (never knew your tummy could have a migraine) and head migraines, he was on a path to healing. The doctor informed me that if he did not start gaining weight, he would do surgery to tighten the esophageal sphincter. I looked the surgery up online. Oh my goodness! This surgery would totally prevent him from vomiting, but could cause terrible stomach pains if he needed to vomit. What? This was not an option that we considered. I did not want him to have even more stomach pains on top of abdominal migraines he already had.

The doctor explained the triggers for a CVS episode. Everything started making sense! Wow! Stress and anxiety is a huge factor. I had to eliminate as much stress as possible for him to grow properly. I made the hard decision to stay at home and homeschool Brady. I was scared at first. Will I teach him enough? Will I get in 175 days of school? Well, Brady made it easy to know I made the right decision. He enjoys learning. He can't handle a large environment and the expectations of teachers. He felt like a failure in public school. He had so many teachers who tried so hard to work with him. There were only a couple that were tough cookies for us. With autism, he needs social interaction. How can he get that if he stays at home? We attend church, so he gets to be with other children and adults there. Once his anxiety was under control, he could function in most places and activities with little issue. He is learning to feel an episode coming on, so we can prevent it. Since I started with home bound school, then homeschool, Brady has become very sociable and eats all the time! It was the hardest decision I think I've ever made to homeschool him. I mean, how was I going to get money to support us?

In life, there's always at least two choices. Each choice has a consequence. I chose to homeschool because it lessened Brady's anxiety, thus reducing his episodes. If I chose to work, I would be bringing home some more money, but I would also still probably be seen as an unreliable employee, and Brady would probably still be so sick. This is the best decision I have made. He is only 11, and is constantly trying to think of "jobs" he can do to earn some money. He is a little worker bee, and I'm proud that he is an overcomer, with no hospitalizations since homeschooling, and only two ER visits. Life is good! So thankful for a CVS diagnosis!

Myths of the Uninvolved Un-schooler
Jamie Martin, editor of Simple Homeschool[7]

I remember the first time I heard the term *unschooling*. I was standing on a street corner chatting with a homeschooling neighbor, who used the term. "What's that?" I asked. While I can't remember her exact definition, I remember my reaction – far from positive. It sounded to me as though unschooling parents ignored their children, not getting really involved in their education.

I knew it wasn't for me since the idea of traditional homeschooling already freaked me out. But then an evolution occurred. And I now find myself parked most resolutely on the informal side of the homeschooling spectrum. I'm not the type who likes being put into a box, so I don't label myself or my family. We pull from a variety of influences in our homeschool and unschooling interest-led learning, Waldorf, and leadership education predominantly. But basically, we just do what works and what best fits our needs.

Last year Jena wrote a post about the two foundational principles of unschooling – that children are born to learn, and that forced learning kills the desire to learn. But what exactly do unschoolers do all day? That varies as much as individual families vary–in other words, a lot! But as I've come to know more unschoolers, it seems to me that we often have in common the following six focuses.

1. *We focus on exposure, not mastery.*
   In my belief, the early years of life (up until age 12 or so) are about allowing my kids to fall in love with learning. I want them

---
[7] See more at: http://simplehomeschool.net/uninvolved-unschooler/#sthash.hnAkwqL1.dpuf

exposed to as much richness and depth as possible. Exposure to language, to words, to writing, to numbers, to art, to music. But I'm not as concerned with the need to master this material according to an artificial timetable, believing instead that mastery will come later as the child's development continues to progress and mature.

2. *We focus on strengths and potential, not weaknesses.*
Few adults have careers based on areas in which they struggled as kids. Typically the most satisfying careers are those with skills in which the person naturally excels and enjoys. Yet in our day-to-day homeschooling it seems so natural to focus on our kids' weaknesses instead of their strengths. Why is that? One day my children will, of course, need to know how to overcome their personal weaknesses. We set the foundation for that when it comes to the area of character development every day. But when it comes to academic achievement, these early years are about building confidence, not pointing out flaws or areas of struggles.

3. *We focus on modeling.*
At my kids' current ages of 8, 7, and 6, I (along with my husband) am the most important influence in their lives. Just as toddlers follow us around wanting to "help" in any way possible, it's only natural for a child to imitate what they see the adults in their life doing. For that reason, I feel my writing career, the books I read, and the example I set to be one of the foundations of my kids' learning. I'm not taking anything away from them by having my own life; instead I'm inspiring them to have their own. My kids know what it means for their parents to have a mission in life, so they know it means they have one, too. Education is all about the process of discovering that mission and becoming equipped to achieve it.

4. *We focus on relationships.*
One thing that unschoolers (and others, of course!) do really well is to focus on relationships. When love flows unconditionally,

not based on whether or not you completed a worksheet correctly, the atmosphere is primed for learning. I have always believed that nurturing is the greatest task I do as a teacher. For this reason cooking and baking with my kids have always been as important as math. When we nurture, defenses go down and everyone opens up to inspiration, ready to tackle new challenges.

5. *We focus on time, not content.*

    Some unschoolers have a spontaneous lifestyle, where there are no set hours for anything and everything is up for negotiation. If that works and makes parents and children happy, I see no problem with it. But it isn't the only way to embrace an interest-learning lifestyle. Our home has a lot of structure because that's what works for us; it's what we need to have a peaceful home. My children know our daily rhythm well, and if you asked them what we do each day, they could quickly run down a litany of activities. But "school" wouldn't be one of them.

    Instead we structure time, not content. I make sure we have plenty of time planned in our day for learning opportunities and one-on-one time. I may even have suggested activities that I think we could work on. But the final choice is up to my kids. I ask, "What do you want to work on today, and how can I help?" I serve as mentor, guide, and friend.

6. *We focus on our conviction and faith in the path we've chosen.*

    It is faith and conviction that enables unschoolers to make choices that place us in the minority of the homeschooling minority. Courage to march to the beat of a completely different cultural drum, to step off the grade level path, challenging and pushing boundaries along the way. I watch my children learn to read without formal lessons. I watch them learn to write and calculate numbers the same way. Not necessarily on my own timetable, but on their own. I listen to their declarations that they love books, they love math, that they can do and be anything.

I marvel at how they are made in God's image, and that even this former perfectionist mama has learned to let go, to trust, and to watch each child blossom in their own perfect and lovely way.

It does a mother's heart good–this releasing, this freedom, this struggle, this joy.

Uninvolved? Hardly. Inspired? Completely.

Schooling Options and Considerations

While some children's school attendance is greatly impacted by CVS, others need only minor adjustments to maintain traditional schooling. Now that my son is seemingly back to a more stable position, we are looking into a Charter School which has more project and creative based learning. Both of these fit his personality more than the traditional school setting. *There are so many options to try for education.*

- Homeschool (parent led)
- Homeschool Co-op (parents and other homeschoolers)
- Homebound (school provides tutors and maintains records)
- Online Schooling (internet based learning)
- Shortened Day /Traditional School with Accommodations (504)
- Traditional School with no accommodations needed
- Private School

Within the public school system of the United State, there are laws in place to ensure a free appropriate education for students with disabilities. There are many options that are available to a parent of a child with a health condition. They may qualify for an Individual Education Plan (IEP) or a 504 which establish accommodations that your child might need within the school setting. When approaching school systems, make sure your child's doctors document the condition and what limitations your child has and how it is likely to affect his or her education. In the United States you can contact the National Learning disability Association for further information. With a well-documented diagnosis of Cyclic Vomiting Syndrome, MOST if not all children with CVS should qualify for a 504 plan mentioned above. The term the school will use is Other Health Impaired. The Individuals with Disabilities Education Act (IDEA) states that:

> **Other health impairment** *means having limited strength, vitality, or alertness, including a heightened alertness to environmental stimuli, that results in limited alertness with respect to the educational environment, that—*
>
> *(i) Is due to chronic or acute health problems such as asthma, attention deficit disorder or attention deficit hyperactivity disorder, diabetes, epilepsy, a heart condition, hemophilia, lead poisoning, leukemia, nephritis, rheumatic fever, sickle cell anemia, and Tourette syndrome; and*
>
> *(ii) Adversely affects a child's educational performance. [§300.8(c)(9)]*

When Health Affects School Attendance

It's not uncommon for a child with an OHI to have periodic absences from school, sometimes even lengthy ones, especially if hospitalization is necessary for whatever reason. During these times, the public school remains responsible for providing educational and related services to the eligible child with OHI. Because IDEA specifically states that special education can be provided in a range of settings, including the home or the hospital, states and school districts will have policies and approaches for addressing children's individualized needs and circumstances.

The school, therefore, is the best source of information about what local policies govern how services are made available to children with OHI who are home-bound or hospitalized. When the child is at home, the school may arrange for a homebound instructor to bring assignments from school to home and help the student complete those assignments. When hospitalized, services may, in fact, be provided by the hospital, through arrangement with the school, although this will vary according to local policies. In any event, the hospital is likely to have policies and procedures of its own, and it's important for the family to find out what they are.

<u>504 Accommodations (as they might relate to CVS kids)</u>

- Reduced Day (more time to adjust to full day or make best use of limited energy if applies)
- Reduction in homework load (to enable kids to be able to get the rest they need and still have a quality life outside of school or extended time to get it done)
- Ability to type if hand weakness is an issue
- Snacks or water throughout the day
- Extended time to work on tests or advanced knowledge of projects so that things get done on time (factoring in the probability of a hospitalization that might disrupt timeline)
- Excused sick days that might be numerous and avoid truancy charges
- Have rest breaks at school as needed
- Open communication between parents and teachers about warning signs of cycles coming
- Make sure school knows what to do if cycle starts at school
- Have plan set up that after x days out school will provide tutor come and help out or help set up peer tutoring
- Get the name of at least one other student in the class for your child to communicate with about assignments

All students' success and positive experiences hinge on excellent parental and teacher communication. Proper health is also a foundational aspect that so many teachers and students take for granted. Education is also about more than test scores and grades. It's about learning and personal growth and achieving skills. Do not let grades or state standards dictate what and when your child must learn. Often a sick child needs to learn how to live with repeated hospital stays, which is both physically and emotionally draining. This can be viewed as a learning experience as well because CVS children do very often become familiar with medical terms and treatments that other kids do not. There's no state standard for that, but it's often a very real part of our children's lives.

Learning is all around us. As parents we need to advocate for our children, and also remember that we are the primary educators. We have the freedom (in most countries) to make decisions of how, where, and what our kids learn. As parents of chronically ill children, we do have to very often get creative in the ways in which this learning happens, and make many sacrifices to see that it happens. We may opt out of public education for a period of time to regain basic health. We may opt for a different style of learning in charter schools. We may opt to stay in public school and fight for tutors and homebound education.

Teachers and educators often have a hard time understanding the cyclic vomiting diagnosis. If your child also has an anxiety disorder they may dismiss or down play the vomiting. Ed Palissamo shared how one time his daughter threw up in school. The teacher now gets it. I know I have sent Andrew's teachers photos of him while he's in the hospital to give them an idea of what a cycle looks like in reality and why we try to avoid them. Currently we are in discussion with the school nurse about giving him the abort medications at school. The suggestion of my being able to drop what I am doing and run to the school and get his medication in the narrow window before he starts vomiting, shows me how little they understand about CVS. And so my role as advocate is never ending. There are so many stories that could be told of the victories and battles CVS parents have with teachers over attendance and assignments. For now it is important to learn your rights, what your options are, and how to advocate better for your child.

There are so many options out there, so it's important not to feel boxed into only one choice. Also remember: this plan can be flexible and change as the needs present themselves. To think differently is not about failing to keep up with the "norm." It's about working with what we have, for the best for our children who live with Cyclic Vomiting Syndrome. Do what's best for the child, even if that means thinking outside of the box. I'd bet we get more than one doctor out of our CVS children, and I'd bet they might be the one to find better treatments options for CVS.

Raising Awareness and Giving Back

Cyclic Vomiting Hits Mainstream Media, Grey's Anatomy
Chandra Wilson

At the 2012 CVSA family conference, I was specifically asked by our sufferers to find a way to get CVS on the television show *Grey's Anatomy*. The show historically focuses less on the medicine of the patients and more on the lives of our regular characters and how they are impacted by the medicine and personal issues.

Still, I made a pitch to my producers for a two episode arc of a 25-year-old male character who repeatedly comes in to the ER with what we know are classic CVS episodes: vomiting bile, writhing in pain, dehydration, and no one there with him to speak as his advocate. He tells of how his school, work, and personal life have been impacted by his illness, and he begs to be taken seriously and for someone to figure out what's wrong. Just as he is about to go through an unnecessary exploratory laparotomy as a last resort to see if something surgical is causing his episodes, he is diagnosed with CVS by Arizona Robbins, who knows of the condition from working in pediatrics.

In response, I was offered "Santa" in a one episode. Weighing the pros and cons, I decided that here was a vehicle to say the name Cyclic Vomiting Syndrome out loud on national television to up to 10 million viewers. Here was an opportunity to produce a Public Service Announcement to drive traffic to CVSA, its message board and

Facebook page. Here was chance that, for all that would be missing in the *Grey's* storyline, your comments and commentaries and posts would fill in the blanks for anyone coming to CVSA for the first time looking for validation or a name to take to their physician or community of support that they never knew existed. We collectively accomplished that the night the episode aired.

Season 9 episode 6 told the story of "Santa", a man who was is taken to the ER and is quickly written off as just someone who had too much to drink and made himself sick, and who does this frequently. However when his lab work come back, it is normal, even the blood alcohol level. Santa then confesses that he has migraines and often turns to drinking to stop the pain of them. The intern doctor then takes the time to help Santa get cleaned up, haircut and all. He looks much better... but is still throwing up on everyone and everywhere. After consulting with another doctor Santa receives the diagnosis of Cyclic Vomiting Syndrome, and given proper medications and a plan to keep the migraines in check.

Phones rang the next morning, hits were made to the website, and comments were posted. Even the disappointed posts spoke graphically of the reasons why the content didn't do enough justice to the experience of CVS. We would need a Television Movie of the Week centered on a family affected by CVS in order to accurately expose what our lives are like as sufferers and caretakers. Maybe I have earned the credibility to accomplish something like that now for us.

Even as I write this, my daughter Sarina has just finished an 11 day stay in Children's Hospital Los Angeles with one of her most violent episodes of relapsing CVS after almost two years of a break. I'm watching for every change in facial expression, keeping the trash can nearby, waiting for her gut to start regular motility again, eager for her normal energy level to return, praying that two days ago was indeed the end of this relapse so that she can go back to being a 19-year-old college student with her whole life in front of her. That's CVS.

Desire to Share the Hope: Joining the CVSA Board of Directors
Tom and Shelley Kupetis

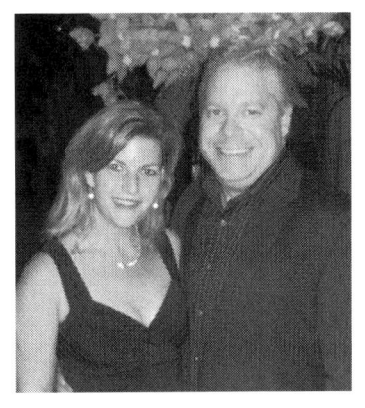

Tom and I joined the CVSA Board of Directors this past summer in August of 2014. We became members of the CVSA five years ago because our 14 year-old daughter, Julia Benway, has been a sufferer the past 10 years. We participated in, and raised funds for, the 2011 and 2013 'Stop the Cycle' 5K Run/Walk in Wisconsin, now known as 'Run for the Bucket'. This is our largest fundraiser of the year that is held annually at the end of May or beginning of June. We also attended the 2012 and 2014 CVSA Adult and Family Conferences to meet other CVS sufferers and families. We wanted to learn more about this rare disease from the medical advisors who attended. We joined the Board to become a part of the growing CVSA family. We are passionate about wanting to help others whose lives have been impacted by CVS, and are now working in Communications and Marketing to grow our membership and raise awareness around the world. We have been very successful in raising funds for the previous walks we attended and look forward to participating again on May 30, 2015. We are committed to raising more money for education and medical research through fundraising events and are hopeful that by providing more valuable information and resources to the public we will greatly improve the quality of life for those afflicted with this disease.

Our volunteer position on the Board these last four months has been such a positive and rewarding experience. Tom and I created our new e-Newsletter 'Highlights' that debuted on October 1st. This members-only benefit is sent out at the beginning of each month, and is designed to help our membership feel more connected to our organization. 'Highlights' features up-to-date news, and provides information on all upcoming fundraising events. We also created our new holiday program called 'Hope Starts Here with Holiday Cheer' for those who would like to make a charitable contribution to the CVSA during the holidays and honor a family member or friend. These donations each year will be used to support operations and our research fund. We are proud to announce and are currently working with the Board of Directors on promoting CVSA International Awareness Day! This inaugural event will take place on March 5, 2015! We are partnering with our sister associations around the world to raise awareness on a worldwide basis and are excited to be a part of this event. Tom and I are proud to be a part of this wonderful organization and are honored to be on the Board of Directors. We will continue to work hard in the future and know in the end that we are truly making a difference in the lives of many children and adult sufferers!

Awareness You Can Wear
Angie Moore

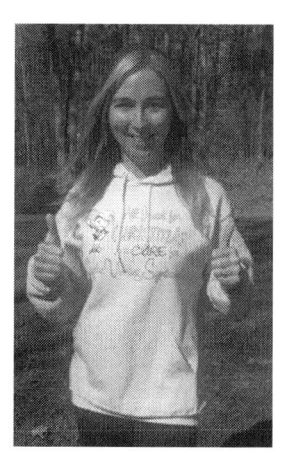

CVS episodes entered my life when I was 25 years old, and was in my last year of veterinarian school. My episodes lasted from 3-5 days, and occurred on a monthly basis. The nausea is intense beyond belief, and never-ending. I vomited anywhere between every 30 seconds to 5 minutes. I spent multiple days hospitalized, and visited Urgent Care centers frequently, seeking relief from my misery. Sometimes I was treated properly, and other times I was treated like a drug-seeker or malingerer. I didn't understand why the physicians weren't interested in why this kept happening to me. They only wanted to give me some medication and send me home, sometimes still sick. I went undiagnosed for 1 ½ years, but finally learned that I have CVS in 2008. Now, finally armed with a name for my illness, I threw myself into researching this disorder obsessively in my spare time.

My greatest resource was the Cyclic Vomiting Syndrome Association. I feel that my journey really began when I found them. I gained valuable information from the website, and eventually became a member so I could use the online community forums called message boards. I began to interact with others who have CVS, and felt validated when others understood and were struggling with the same issues that I was. I also learned the treatments and medications that have helped me since then. The message boards became like a second family to me. Eight years later, I still have episodes, but they are less frequent and much less intense than they used to be. The message boards have helped me through the most difficult part of my life that I have faced so far. I have made life-long friends many people there.

In June 2014 I attended the CVSA Conference in Milwaukee, WI. It was a life-changing experience. I met Dr. Venkatesen, who agreed to take my case. She saw me as a patient in October 2014, and I am thankful to finally have a doctor who knows more about CVS than I do! The conference provided me a lot of information, and a lot of motivation. I was inspired by the people who run the organization and gave the presentations, and decided that I wanted to give back to CVSA since they have helped me so much. I was asked to join the fundraising committee for CVSA and accepted with enthusiasm.

I've been working on promoting awareness of CVS via t-shirts. A company called Booster.com (aka Custom Ink) provides the means for me to create any design on shirts. Once I design the shirt, we advertise it through the CVSA online community. If we make the minimum order, the company sends the shirts to print, and then ships them to everyone who ordered them. CVSA gets a percentage of the sales from the shirt, plus any extra donations people choose to make.

The first shirt was the "Cyclic Vomiting Warrior" shirt. We sold 136 shirts and raised $1243.89 for the CVSA! Our most recent campaign was the "All I Want For Christmas is a Cure For CVS" shirts. We sold 150 shirts and raised a total of $1036.38! Our next campaign will be in February and will be a shirt dedicated to the theme of CVS International Day, which is on March 5th, 2015. The shirts have been a lot of fun to design and are a great way to promote awareness of our disorder in our communities. I am truly grateful for the opportunity to give back to CVSA since it has given me so much. Every day is a new day, and my goal is to learn new ways to live with and treat CVS, as well as to help others do the same.

Using the Cuteness Factor: Trinity's Troops
Tiffany Sharp

Trinity's Troops is a Facebook page I started when a post about my daughter Trinity (who has CVS) went viral. I posted a collage of her when she was in hospitals and just wrote a little bit about what she goes through. I just wanted to get my frustrations out about our daily battle. Little did I know it would blow up so quickly! I woke up the next day with hundreds of friend requests and that's when Trinity's Troops was born. I have had an overabundance of support and now we are at over 10,600 likes and still growing! All I wanted to do was be a voice for my daughter and now we don't feel so alone. To all of the parents going through this, it doesn't define our children. It may make them grow up a little quicker than they have to, but they can do anything. We have to reassure our children that it's not about the illness, it's about them. We do giveaways for bumper stickers for Trinity's Troops and we also have raised money with shirt sales.

Better Late Than Not At All, a Pumpkin Says It All
Amy Beaudion

My name is Amy and I have a wonderful husband and three kids. As a child I was sick, a lot! We noticed that if I was up late I would get really sick for a day or two...if I was stressed or anxious about anything, I'd be sick for days. The doctors kept telling is it was the flu — because apparently having the flu about 10 times a year was normal?

Starting in 7th grade I was homeschooled till I graduated in 2000. I hadn't had nearly as many episodes as earlier years so thought that maybe I outgrew whatever it was. I attempted traditional college but ended up dropping out as my episodes came back with a vengeance. Through three pregnancies, the first and last had me on bed rest and home IV treatment due to what they said was Hyperemesis.

Finally, in late 2009 my new primary care reviewed my medical records and advised me to see a GI doctor as he felt I had CVS. Many tests later I was finally diagnosed in early 2010. My diagnosing physician unfortunately passed in 2012 so I was transferred another doctor in the practice. He was pretty unfamiliar with CVS and more testing showed I also have Gastroparesis. He determined at that point that he wouldn't be able to treat me due to his unfamiliarity, and referred me to an expert in Boston who has been amazing since I began seeing him, although my cycles are still frequent, lengthy, and painful. I lost my jobs while I was hospitalized out of state in Boston.

My family and I made this pumpkin to raise awareness.

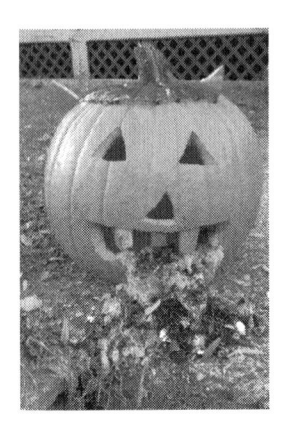

Racing Towards Awareness at the Boston Marathon
Denise Kaplan

Rob Cook was a first time Boston Marathoner for 2014. He ran in support of those who live with Cyclic Vomiting Syndrome (CVS). After the events of the 2013 Boston Marathon, Rob decided he really wanted to be part of that race, but had no ties to CVS. Rob started working at Genzyme as an intern and then continued on as an employee with them. As an adult, working in the field of rare diseases is all he has ever done. Interestingly enough though, he had never heard of CVS before.

Genzyme's Running For Rare Diseases team has many runners raising awareness and fundraising for various different rare diseases. The National Organization of Rare Disorders (NORD) helps support individuals with the hundreds of rare disorders in the United States, with participation in treatments and research. Rob set a lofty goal to raise $2500 for NORD in the 2014 Boston Marathon when he joined the team, and then simply began running!

It was by chance that Rob learned of Patrick, and Patrick became his Patient Partner. The Running for Rare Diseases team members are all typically linked up with a patient with a rare disorder. It is a great way to raise awareness, to build hope and relationships, and to raise money for research and treatments. Rob and Patrick's connection was forged after a social media post by Patrick's mother! Through discussions about CVS with a friend over social media, a connection was formed with Genzyme's Running for Rare Diseases team, then with NORD, and then ultimately with Rob.

After a few telephone calls it was clear: Although it was a match that seemed to be made by chance, it was a perfect one that ultimately appeared as if it were meant to be. Patrick is an 8 year-old boy from Colorado who has been suffering from CVS practically since birth. Although he is very bright, he struggles to physically and emotionally keep up with his recreational interests and school needs. Despite the huge discrepancies in age, geographical location, and health status, Patrick and Rob shared a lot of common interests: they both enjoy sports (including Boston Bruins hockey and Red Sox baseball), music, and a belief in living life to its fullest.

Rob puts his heart and soul into everything he sets out to do. He took on the role of Partner to Patrick in that very way, listening to stories about his active lifestyle and about his limitations with having CVS. Rob has been helpful in lending some positive outlooks, expressing common interests and in motivation for Patrick to keep working through the tough times. He became a role model for persevering through difficult tasks...The very reason Rob set out to run the Boston Marathon in the first place!

Through this process of being matched for the Marathon, realizations have been made by both Rob and Patrick that people are trying to make a difference in the lives of those with rare disorders, that CVS is real and can be quite challenging to live with (especially for young, active children), and also that "total strangers" can be immensely motivational and form bonds that are life altering!

Rob and Patrick were Patient Partners in the 2014 Boston Marathon, but Rob ran for hundreds and even possibly thousands of others who have CVS on April 21, 2014. He was cheered on by many during the grueling 26.2 mile route, including one very loud and grateful 8 year-old!

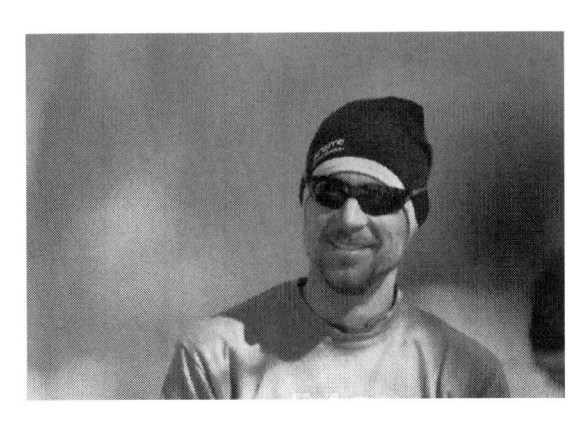

Cyclic Vomiting Syndrome New Zealand
Dynelle Smallwood

My daughter Bayley was first diagnosed with CVS at age 8 with episodes every 9 days. I was relieved to have an answer. The specialist prescribed daily medication, and I assumed that would be all we needed. Bayley would be fine now. 102 days later she was sick again, then 108 days later sick again. What was going on? I thought we had solved it. I needed more information, more support.

I found an online support group on Facebook. I now had tons of support from parents going through the same things. They taught me about abort drugs, the mito connection, and just how lucky I was. Only they were all overseas and the drugs that were working for them all had different names. I wanted some support from New Zealand. I wanted to know if anyone else from our little country was going through this too. I wanted to know if they had found a doctor who knew more about CVS, and I wanted to know what the drugs were called here.

It wasn't until I had seen other parents posting on Facebook, asking if anyone else was from Ireland or Australia and then seeing that they had found a Facebook group for their country, that I realised that maybe to find these answers I would have to start a group for NZ myself. So I created a Facebook group called Cyclic Vomiting Syndrome New Zealand with the hope of finding others from New Zealand who could share their experiences and information. Maybe they would have questions too and maybe I could share what I have learnt. I contacted CVSA and told them about the group and they added it to their list of International Support Groups and also sent me their information pack.

I figure we will be in this for quite some time yet so we may as well make the most of our situation and find something good to share. Now I just have to get the word out there and find some more members.

A Novel Approach Breaking the Cycle
Tricia Anderson

I never expected my little girl to have to fight a battle with a foe she couldn't see. At the age of one, she did. Ali was thirteen months when her first horrific vomiting episode started. After a day and a half of throwing up off and on she had to be admitted to the hospital. She was so dehydrated that the only vein they could put the IV in was in her forehead. I hated seeing her like that as I held her on my chest. We watched the rest of those that were around her waiting for the stomach bug to appear. No one else was sick. It seemed odd she was the only one.

The vomiting episodes didn't go away. In fact, they came back every three weeks like clockwork. During the days in between each episode she would watch the other kids in daycare play, too weak to get up and join them. She wore clothes out before she outgrew them. My battles are nothing compared to hers.

Every time Ali was in an episode, I was on the phone with the doctor. I received the same answer every time. It's a virus. After about six months of my constant phone calls, the doctor was at her wits end with me admitting it could be something other than a virus. She mentioned Cyclic Vomiting Syndrome (CVS). I ran with it like a dog with a bone.

I asked every gastroenterologist I could think of about it. I finally e-mailed the head of pediatrics gastroenterology at the University of Iowa Hospitals and Clinics and asked if my daughter's symptoms could be CVS. He responded that he wanted to see her immediately. We made the appointment, he ran the tests, and it was confirmed – my now two-year-old daughter had CVS. The bad news – since she was so young he didn't know of any treatment. He prescribed medicine without the assurance it would work.

In the meantime I researched CVS. I found the Cyclic Vomiting Syndrome Association website. I also discovered that the expert in pediatric CVS, Dr. B.U.K Li, was at that time in Chicago. I asked the GI doctor at UIHC if we could get a referral. He was delighted. Two weeks later, Ali was seeing Dr. Li and she was put on the correct medications. Within the month she was playing, laughing and growing just like any other normal child.

Today Ali is eleven. She plays volleyball and basketball. She loves learning programming for her school's First Lego League robot. She is sassy, beautiful and funny. And she still has CVS. She takes daily medication to control it. She has a special Zofran creme she can put on her wrists to stop an episode. She has been hospitalized six times. Her older brothers, father, and I have all her rituals down to a science.

Along with being Ali's mom, I am a romance and children's author. When I received my first contract ever with a publisher, my first thought was to "do good." Being a published author and knowing other people were reading my work was literally my greatest dream come true. I wanted to share my incredible gift by doing something with my talent. I just wasn't sure how.

The contract arrived during Ali's first basketball season. We learned all sorts of new things about her CVS while she played. If she ran too much, played too hard and overheated, she started into an episode. However, just like her mother, Ali is very stubborn. She would play no matter what. We invested in an ice vest from Amazon and used quite a bit of Dr. Li's crème. She looked like a linebacker with the vest and all those ice packs on but she played.

Going through all this with Ali and her basketball answered my urge to "do good." The idea was crazy but I was excited to do it. I was going to write a romance novel about a woman who had CVS but didn't know it and a hero who would sacrifice to find her diagnosis. Would anyone read it? Probably not. Who would want to read a book about a woman who constantly vomited? The process was slow since I had two novels that were contracted to be written.

The process of writing the book put me in contact with countless people who I can't thank enough. The CVSA put me in touch with a couple adult CVS sufferers, Silvia Robey and Marie Pierce, who guided me through what it was like to be an adult living with it. Finally in September 2013 I submitted the book, *Breaking the Cycle*, to my publisher. I wasn't sure they would take it. Vomiting was an uncomfortable subject. They were in the business of selling books. Could it even possibly sell? I waited anxiously for an answer and I didn't have to wait long. Within a week I had the contract for *Breaking the Cycle*.

Breaking the Cycle was already the #1 best seller on the Sweet Cravings website when it released on January 13th, 2014. Since then it's been on the Amazon Top 100 Bestsellers list for Sports Fiction in both the US and UK multiple times and has won the April Ind'tale Crème de la Cover contest. To me, the accolades do not matter. Making more people aware of CVS was my only goal. Multiple readers have mentioned they never knew about Cyclic Vomiting Syndrome and went to the CVSA website to learn more. The word is spreading. I am excited that *Breaking the Cycle* is doing the good it was meant to.

The Sky's the Limit for CVS Kids

■ ■ ■

CVS kids very often appreciate of finding the joys of every day. Still, they suffer in ways most children never experience. They lose days to vomiting and miss out on numerous events and special occasions. CVS can be very unpredictable throughout the course of one's life. Sometime the preventative medications work, and other times they do not. We hold the good times close to our hearts as special memories, when we finally have found a treatment plan that is working more often than not. These "breaks" and successes give us hope that CVS will not ALWAYS control our lives.

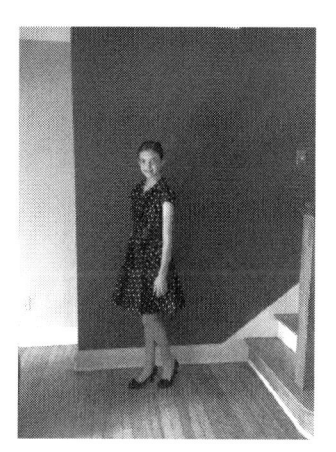

Despite having this disorder I run cross country, I sing for two Catholic Churches, and I play the piano. I continue to be on the Dean's List at school and I thank my parents for always being so supportive and helping me do so well in school. It is very hard living with Cyclic Vomiting Syndrome because you never know when it's going to strike. I refuse to let it stop me from all the things I enjoy, but I do worry when that seven week mark is approaching. This disorder is real and it's no fun.

— Brianna, age 12

CVS kids do things in their own way. They come to appreciate simple victories that others overlook:

I have been waiting all year to go to outdoor school! I knew I might only make it a day but I just wanted to go. I had an episode the Sunday before leaving, so I thought I got it out of my system. Camp was amazing. I had so much fun playing outside while learning new things. The food was amazing. We got dessert at lunch and dinner. I met new friends and learned campfire songs. I was a little worried about getting sick in front of people but I have learned to "swallow" and excuse myself.

Day 1, nothing, day 2 another sunny day in the high 70's, day 3 going good playing and learning. Day 4 water activities my favorite part! Then - BAM! It starts. I puke just before snack time. The counselor asked "is this what I think it is?" I reply yep! Just like that I know my outdoor school trip is over, but I was so happy to have made it four days! I walk to the nurse get a bucket and call my mom to come pick me up. I know the routine: laying down, waiting to go to the ER for IV meds, and treatment for dehydration. I know CVS sucks put I always try to look for something positive. Making it four days at outdoor school was the best!

— Lyndsey age 11

There are many other simple joys that that we as a community of parents feel, such pride and joy when one of our own is able to enjoy special events and not have CVS steal the day from us. Such as how Sean made it to his cotillion with his friends this year, and is back in school for part of the day. Also how Ashten is finally returning to school full time after being homebound for most of his first grade year. Andrew will now be strong enough to return to a group learning environment. Millie has managed to do all of her GCES exams, with only one episode, we wait with bated breath every month hoping and praying! CVS has been kind to us this month. Hoping she gets to her prom coming up. Despite all his absences, Jett still made the A honor roll and is in accelerated classes. He is involved with community outreach and just has a great heart. While he struggles sometimes, he has managed not to let CVS define who he is.

Alexis made her First Communion with her class after her mom worked tirelessly to educate the priests in her area about how CVS impacted her daughter.

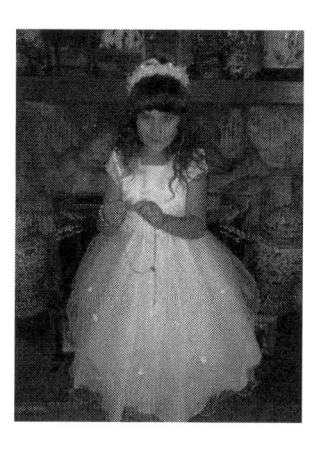

Beth seems to have finally made it to the other side, and her CVS is no longer controlling her life as it once had. Her mother proudly shared with me that:

> The worst years of our CVS journey are becoming a faded and distant memory. When I see a picture or video of Beth between 7 and 10 years of age, the memories and the strong emotions attached to them quickly come back. CVS dominated our life during that time. But for right now, it isn't that big of a deal. At age 12, it's still with us, but the episodes are very infrequent with less intense symptoms that only last part of a day. Dr. Li predicted that things may change for the better after menstruation cycles start, and he was right.

I still worry about the next episode and whether or not it might steal a good memory by interfering with some fun plans or a big event that can't be rescheduled. But I no longer go to bed every night with a desperate prayer for help. I know CVS will always be with us, but for right now, it's manageable. Having been through what seemed like the worst nightmare possible for 3+ years, "manageable" is a great place to be.

I am once again scheduling family vacation plans and allowing Beth to be involved in all of her favorite activities without intense fear of disappointment and frustration. I never imagined that an "almost normal" life could be so wonderful! So when the next episode hits and your child is miserable, please tell him or her that you know things WILL get better and believe it. We all have different CVS stories, but we can all share the same faith for a better tomorrow for our kids. I know it's tough (believe me I know), but I hope our story will help strengthen your faith and give you a little more coping power until the CVS nightmare becomes a distant memory for you as well!

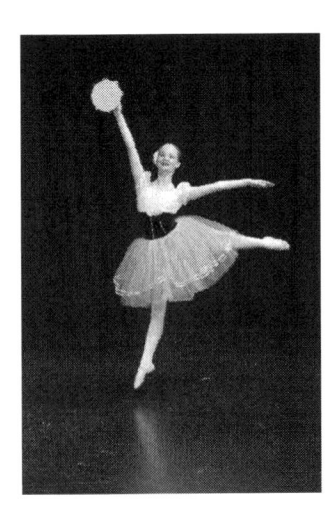

Leonie happily dancing

Leonie had a solo dance competition on the day of her 16th birthday. She woke feeling nauseous and spent the day in bed. Half an hour before the family was ready to leave for the comps she was in bed in tears. Her mother told her she didn't have to dance but she did not want to let CVS win and off she went to the competitions. Leonie's dance friends helped do her hair and makeup and were a great support to her get on stage. There was no prize from the adjudicator that night but anyone who knew what she was dealing with would have given her 1st prize.

Last summer Mia competed in the Gothia Cup in Gothenberg, Sweden, the world's largest youth soccer tournament. She played more than 10 games over a four day period and spent three more days training with professional coaches at FCN Denmark. Different time zone, different food, lack of sleep and lots of exercise and still no episode!

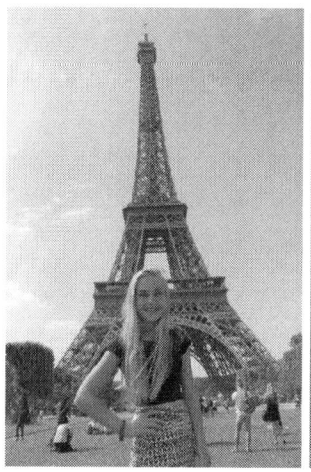

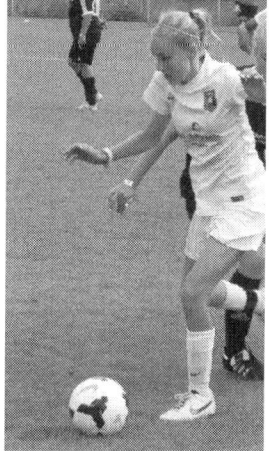

CVS is an awful condition, but if we are able to look at it from a different standpoint, we will be able to get more out of what life has to offer us. If we view it, not as the enemy to be attacked, but rather as a bodily response that you can learn to live with, you will conserve your energy for things you and your child really want to do. When I say live with it, I mean learn how to manage it, offering supportive therapy when needed. This is not meant as "suck it up buttercup" as many people might write it off as.

Each day the medical community learns more and more about CVS. Just 20 years ago most children went undiagnosed. Now we have options even if there is no cure. This should give us hope. Connie Kelly shares that "a working treatment plan is close to a cure in my eyes…keep the faith. No one knows the future of the medical discoveries with illness…look how far the world has come with other illnesses." We should not give up hope.

We as CVS parents are proud of our kids. We rejoice in simple things that many others take for granted. We know the struggles they have overcome and the things they have missed out on because of them. We stand strong, cheering them on, reminding them that it's not always going to be like this. They are only limited by what they choose. The severity and treatment path varies from person to person. We each choose our own path that may be different from others, but that's ok. We seek out the correct path for our family at the time. That path has many twists and turns as we go through life. There are mild years, and years that we'd rather forget. But we never ever give up, we are strong and lean on each other to make it through.

Want to know what a CVS child can do? Anything they set their mind to. I am a CVS child, now grown. Researching and writing a book like this one is possible despite my missing 75% of my first grade year in school to CVS (50% of 7th grade for similar reasons as well). I was able to graduate high school, college, and graduate school. My mom was told "she will never graduate high school" by my first grade teacher. I proved them all wrong. With the publishing of this book, I am reaching out to others like myself so that they might know they are not alone. Being a CVS kid turned CVS parent, I've had the pain of seeing cyclic vomiting from both sides and want to world to know that CVS is real. It will challenge your family in any way it can but always remember that with support, the sky is the limit for today's and tomorrow's CVS kids.

Appendix

Cyclic Vomiting Syndrome Association (CVSA) December 2014

CVSA USA/Canada is a non-profit disease association, founded in 1993. This organization was founded by a handful of parents, patients and professionals and has grown steadily in numbers, awareness and impact. Cyclic Vomiting Syndrome is an uncommon, unexplained disorder of children and some adults that was first described by Dr. Samuel Gee in 1882. The condition is characterized by recurrent, prolonged attacks of severe nausea, vomiting and prostration with no apparent cause. Vomiting occurs at frequent intervals (5-10 times an hour at the peak) for hours to 10 days (1-4 most commonly). The episodes tend to be similar to each other in symptoms and duration and are self-limited. The person is typically well between episodes.

Up until 1993 very little had been written about CVS and many patients and families suffered in a realm of isolation. In 1998, Dr. Richard Boles, M.D. was invited to present his early research at the 2nd International Scientific Symposium on CVS at the Medical College of Wisconsin in Milwaukee. Since that time, Dr. Boles has become one of CVSA's primary medical advisors and has brought a great deal of research and resulting information to the CVSA membership and medical advisors. This information links CVS with mitochondrial disease.

The focus of our early years was to aggressively seek out patients and families in order to offer peer support. Now we offer a newsletter three times a year, an active message board and facebook page, call-in support groups, volumes of replies to inquiries, doctor referral, just to name some of our patient support programs. Equally important has been our effort to educate professionals about this illness, its diagnosis and treatment. Both of these efforts have been effective and ongoing. CVSA has also been able to realize a 3rd mission of supporting research with funding, logistical support and co-investigators.

There are seven CVSA associations around the world. Australia, Denmark, Italy, Japan, Spain, United Kingdom and CVSA USA/Canada. In addition to the associations, there are contact families and/or physicians in 33 countries. CVSA International has an informal network of education, support and research work loosely governed by a set of written guidelines. CVSA USA/Canada is governed by a volunteer lay Board of Directors and well advised by the multi-specialty Professional Advisory Board.

CVSA International has sponsored two international scientific symposia on CVS - London 1994 and Milwaukee, Wisconsin 1998. Funding has been provided by membership families, foundations and corporations. The 1998 symposium was funded largely by a Workshop/Conference Grant from the NIH (NIDDK, NINDS, Office of Rare Disorders). There have been multiple brainstorming scientific/research meeting over the years as well. These unusually successful multi-specialty meetings have resulted in a number of proposed collaborative research efforts and publications. Proceedings of both symposia have been published as supplements to reputable peer-reviewed journals primarily through family funding efforts. CVSA has hosted ten bi-annual family/patient conferences as well. Scientific activity continues mostly with the CVSA Primary Medical Advisors. Our current scientific work includes collaboration and financial support for the 1st Bi-Annual Conference on the Biology and Control of Nausea and Vomiting - 2013. Dr. Charles Horn, PhD of the University of Pittsburgh is the co-organizer and a medical advisor on CVSA. CVSA has a larger part to play in the upcoming 2015 conference. We are also starting work toward co-sponsorship of an effort to develop treatment guidelines or a consensus statement on the diagnosis and management of CVS in adults.

In October of 2010, CVSA was contacted by actress, Chandra Wilson – Dr. Bailey of *Grey's Anatomy*. Chandra's daughter has CVS and mitochondrial disease and is a patient of Dr. Boles. After developing a working relationship, Chandra agreed to be the national spokesperson for CVSA. Her media activity on our behalf has taken CVSA to a new level of awareness. Chandra and her daughter attended and did the keynote presentation at our 10th International Family/Patient conference. She also attended the simultaneous scientific conference. Thanks to Chandra, in November of 2012, an episode of *Grey's Anatomy* featured a patient with CVS. This airing resulted in over 700 calls and emails to the CVSA office and new found help for many of these CVSA continues with dogged determination to reach out with support and education to patients, families and professionals who are still affected by CVS and trying to cope in isolation.

Kathleen Adams, BSN, RN
President, Co-founder, Research Liaison

Extreme Emesis: Cyclic Vomiting Syndrome

by Narayanan Venkatasubramani, Thangam Venkatesan and BU. K. Li

Reprinted with Permission from Practical Gastroenterology, September 2007

Cyclic vomiting syndrome (CVS) is an idiopathic disorder that has been primarily identified in children but has recently been increasingly recognized in adults. Acute episodes are typically misdiagnosed as gastroenteritis and food poisoning that leads to a three-to-eight year delay in diagnosis. The major challenge for the frontline clinician is to differentiate CVS, a functional disorder without laboratory markers, from the myriad organic causes of vomiting. Better awareness and earlier recognition and treatment of CVS will reduce the morbidity, avoid unnecessary investigations and repeated hospitalizations that are estimated to incur $17,035 per patient annually (1). This article focuses on the clinical features, including differences between adults and children, potential pathophysiologic mechanisms, pertinent exclusionary investigations and specific treatment approaches.

Cyclic vomiting syndrome was first described by Samuel Gee in 1882 (2) and named cyclic vomiting by Smith in 1937 (3). CVS is characterized by recurrent, sudden, stereotypical, disabling, discrete episodes of intense nausea and vomiting that can last a few hours to days interspersed with varying weeks of symptom-free intervals.

EPIDEMIOLOGY

The estimated prevalence of CVS in children is in the range of 0.3%–2.2 % (4). This disorder is primarily recognized in children, primarily Caucasians (mean age of onset at five years), with increasing recognition in adults (mean age of onset at 35 years). There have been case reports of symptoms starting as early as the sixth day of life and as late as 73 years. In children, females appear to be more affected than males, com-pared to a male predominance in adults (5,6).

CVS is now considered to be a functional brain-gut disorder in which central signals initiate a peripheral gastrointestinal manifestation—vomiting. There appear to be a number of host susceptibility factors including a family member with migraine headaches (82% of CVS versus 14% of chronic vomiting patients), mitochondrial dysfunction, and autonomic dysregulation. There is a strong matrilineal inheritance of CVS from migraines, elevated lactic acid, and several heteroplasmies in the control region of the mtDNA supporting involvement of mtDNA (7,8). There is also heightened sympathetic cardiovascular tone in children with CVS compared to controls (9,10).

These factors taken together suggest that inadequate cellular energy production at times of heightened needs (trigger factors mentioned below) leads to a metabolic crisis. This in turn leads to a deleterious effect on high energy requiring autonomic neurons resulting in an episodic autonomic crisis with vomiting. Similar to migraines, there appear to be common triggering factors including psychological stress (especially excitement) and infections. Based largely on extensive animal studies, Taché, et al have proposed that the hypothalamic secretion of corticotrophin-releasing factor (CRF) could act as the neuroendocrine trigger of vomiting (11). CRF stimulates the inhibitory fibers of the dorsal motor nucleus of the vagus decreasing the upper GI tract motility (and potentially triggers vomiting). By also acting on the locus ceruleus, CRF also increases sympathetic tone and the associated signs of pallor, flushing, fever, lethargy, excess salivation, and diarrhea.

CYCLIC VERSUS CHRONIC PATTERNS OF RECURRENT VOMITING

The key to diagnosis of CVS is recognition of the cyclic pattern of these repeated vomiting episodes. Recurrent vomiting can be divided into two temporal patterns described as either cyclic or chronic (Table 1). The cyclic pattern is highly supportive of an eventual diagnosis of CVS, once the radiographic, laboratory and endoscopic evaluations are negative. The chronic pattern usually indicates a disorder such as gastroesophageal reflux or gastritis within the upper GI tract (12). It is also important to recognize that CVS is but one of the causes of a cyclic vomiting pattern. Other causes of severe episodic vomiting in children include surgical lesion (malrotation with intermittent volvulus), metabolic (acute intermittent porphyria) and endocrine disorders (Addison disease) (13). CVS is frequently misdiagnosed in emergency departments as rotavirus gastroenteritis and food poisoning; however patients with CVS are qualitatively (pallor, listlessness) and quantitatively (more likely to require IV rehydration) sicker (6) than patients with rotavirus infections.

Table 1
Difference Between Chronic and Cyclical Pattern of Vomiting

	Cyclic or Epidsodic	Chronic
Intensity of vomiting	High (≥4 emesis/hour at the peak)	Low (1–2 emesis/hour)
Frequency of vomiting	Low (1–2 episodes/month)	Nearly daily
Diagnoses	Highly supportive of CVS or disorders outside the GI tract (e.g., hydroenephrosis)	GERD or gastritis (disorders of the upper GI tract)
Dehydration	Common	Uncommon

DIAGNOSTIC CRITERIA

CVS is currently defined by fulfilling "essential and supportive" criteria. The Consensus diagnostic criteria for CVS in children (14) and adults (15) are shown in Table 2A and 2B.

Table 2A
Consensus Diagnostic Criteria in Children

Essential criteria
- Recurrent, severe, discrete episodes of vomiting
- Varying intervals of normal health between episodes
- Duration of vomiting episodes from hours to days
- No apparent cause of vomiting (negative laboratory, radiographic and endoscopic testing)

Supportive criteria
- Pattern
  - Stereotypical: each episode similar as to time of onset, intensity, duration, symptoms and signs within individuals
  - Self-limited: episodes resolve if left untreated
- Associated symptoms
  - Nausea, abdominal pain, headache, motion sickness, photophobia, and lethargy
- Associated signs
  - Pallor, dehydration, fever, excess salivation and social withdrawal

Table 2B
Diagnostic Criteria* in Adults

- Must include all of the following
  - Stereotypical episodes of vomiting regarding onset (acute) and duration (less than one week)
  - Three or more discrete episodes in the prior year
  - Absence of nausea and vomiting between episodes
- Supportive criterion
  - History or family history of migraine headaches

*Criteria fulfilled for the last three months with symptom onset at least six months before diagnosis

CLINICAL FEATURES

Typical CVS episodes tend to have a stereotypic pat-tern within individuals and can be subdivided into four phases (16). The initial prodromal phase before the onset of vomiting often begins suddenly with symptoms of nausea, sweating, abdominal pain, irritability and anorexia. However, they usually do not have visual symptoms of typical migraine aura. The prodrome is often brief and rapidly progresses to vomiting within one-to-two hours. The second phase is the emetic phase characterized by relentless nausea and vomiting and persistence of the prodromal symptoms. The unique rapid fire (often every five-to-ten minutes) vomiting often begins early in the morning between 2–4 A.M. or upon awakening at 7 A.M., although in some episodes start later. The vomiting episodes last for one-to-three days in children and six-to-nine days in adults (17,18).

Symptoms of anxiety and panic attacks appear to be common in adults during the first two phases. The patient may be so listless as to appear in a coma-like state, unable to ambulate or speak. The third phase is the recovery phase which begins with the disappearance of nausea and vomiting to the point of return of near normal appetite and activity. This may be brief, like the prodromal phase, so that the patient appears to suddenly awaken like "turning off a switch" and be able to eat within one-to-two hours of cessation of emesis. The fourth phase is the well-interval phase during which the patient is symptom-free. In children, there may be four weeks to several months of normal health. This differs from adult patients in whom some 50% have significant symptoms, usually dyspeptic nausea and/or sporadic vomiting in between. This has been called coalescence of episodes. Recent studies indicate that 70% of adult patients have psychological co-morbidities and a previous diagnosis of or features characteristic of, one or more of the following: anxiety (63%–84%), panic attacks (68%), depression (78%), alcoholism and/or drug abuse (5,16). An unpublished report in children estimates a high prevalence of anxiety (39%) and mood symptoms in children compared to norms of the Children's Symptom

Inventory and population normal for internalizing psychiatric disorders (Dr. Sally Tarbell)

OTHER FEATURES

Some patients complain of intense abdominal pain requiring narcotics for relief and/or severe headaches. Others may present with low-grade fever, vomiting, and diarrhea that is easily confused with acute viral gastroenteritis. Hypertension with tachycardia has also been observed in a subgroup with a more severe (pro-longed) variant of CVS described by Sato, et al (19,20). The intense nausea experienced during the emetic phase of CVS has induced behaviors that have been mistakenly considered bulimic or psychotic. For example, intense thirst has been reported in some adult patients drinking as much as 14 liters of water in a day, yet this has been described by patients to attenuate the nausea. Dehydration with electrolyte abnormalities ($-Na+, -K+, O2$), hypoglycemia, and gastrointestinal bleeding secondary to prolapse gastropathy, Mallory-Weiss tear or esophagitis are some of the frequent complications of CVS. The main differences between adult and children with cyclic vomiting syndrome are shown in Table 3.

PRECIPITATING FACTORS

Two-thirds of families are able to identify events that appear to precipitate a child's episode (21–23). The two most common triggers are infections of any kind (31%), particularly chronic sinusitis, and stress (47%) at school or home. Interestingly, the most common scenario was positive excitement that included birth-days, holidays and family reunions. The most frequent triggers in adults are menstrual periods, noxious stress, pleasant excitement and fatigue.

Table 3
Comparison of CVS Clinical Features Between Children and Adults

	Children (Li/Balint)	Adults (Fleisher/Namin)
Age of onset	4.8 years (earliest: 6 days)	30–35 years (oldest: 73 years)
Delay in diagnosis	2.6 years	8 years
Female:Male	57:43	30:42
Episodes pattern		
Frequency	every 2–4 weeks	every 3 months
Duration (range)	1–2 days (1–10)	4–6 days (1–21)
Periodicity	49%	not reported
Early A.M. onset	42%	50%
Stereotypical	99%	85%
Prodrome	72%, 1.5 hours	93%
Symptoms	nausea, anorexia, pallor	nausea, epigastric pain
Recovery to oral feeding	6 hours	24 hours, 10 days
Relieving factors	deep sleep	hot bath/shower (56%–72%)
Precipitating factors	stress (47%), infection (31%)	stress (50%), menses
Co-morbid conditions	anxiety	anxiety, panic attacks, migraine, depression
Inter-episodic nausea	<6%	63%
Coalescence of episodes	few	50%
Symptoms		
Vomiting	6 times/hr at peak, bile (81%)	8.5 times/hr, bile
Systemic	pallor, salivation, listlessness,	intense thirst (33%)
GI	anorexia, nausea, diarrhea, abdominal pain	abdominal pain, diarrhea
Neurologic	headache, photophobia, phonophobia, vertigo	irritable, confused
Natural history	3.6 years 28+% progress to migraine	5.2 years
FH of migraine	82%	23%–57%
Complications	dehydration, esophagitis	dehydration, esophagitis, laprotomy (18%)
Morbidity	14–25 days of missed school/year	32% completely disabled before initiating therapy

NATURAL HISTORY

In children, CVS often resolves by early puberty. Approximately 28% of patients with CVS have migraine onset at 9.5 years and it is projected that 75% will develop migraines by age 18. In a cross-sectional school survey by Abu-Arafeh and Russell, the mean respective ages of children with CVS, abdominal migraine, and migraine headaches are 5.3, 10.3 and 11.5 years suggesting a sequential progression among the three entities (24). Although some do experience all three phases, most children with CVS develop migraine headaches without passing through an intervening abdominal migraine stage. In a series of 41 adult patients studied by Fleisher, the natural history differed substantially from that in children as nearly half of the adult patients experienced deterioration over time either by the coalescence of episodes or development of chronic inter-episodic dyspeptic nausea. One-third of adults were completely disabled and required financial support at the time of initial consultation before therapy was initiated (16).

DIFFERENTIAL DIAGNOSIS

The major challenge is to differentiate CVS, a functional disorder from the myriad organic causes of vomiting. Although the cyclic vomiting pattern usually indicates the diagnosis of cyclic vomiting syndrome in 88%, approximately 12% of children who presented with the typical cyclic pattern were found to have a specific, underlying cause for their vomiting (Table 4). The differential diagnosis is broad both in children and adults. Since structural and metabolic conditions typically pre-sent in childhood, especially acute hydronephrosis and malrotation with volvulus, more extensive testing for renal, GI, intracranial, metabolic and endocrine disorders has been applied to children (25).

Table 4
Differential Diagnosis of Cyclic Vomiting Pattern by Relative Frequency

		Children	Adults
Gastrointestinal	Inflammatory bowel disease	+	++
	Malrotation with volvulus	+++	+
	Chronic intestinal pseudo-obstruction	+	++
	Partial intestinal obstruction	+	++
	Neoplasms	−	+
	Cholelithiasis	+	++
	Recurrent pancreatitis	+	++
Genitourinary	Hydronephrosis 2° UPJ obstruction (Dietl crisis)	+++	−
	Nephrolithiasis	+	+
Central nervous system	Hydrocephalus	+	+
	Arnold-Chiari malformation	++	−
	Subtentorial neoplasm	+	−
	Familial dysautonomia	+	−
Metabolic	Disorders of fatty acid oxidation	+	−
	Acute intermittent porphyria	+	++
	Urea cycle defects	+	−
	Mitochondrial disorders	+++	−
Endocrine	Addison disease	+	+
	Pheochromocytoma	+	+
	Diabetic gastroparesis	+	++
Psychological	Munchausen syndrome-by-proxy	+	−
Other	Pregnancy	+	+
	Drugs and medication	−	++

DIAGNOSTIC INVESTIGATIONS

To date, how much exclusionary testing should be per-formed in patients with the cyclic vomiting pattern is unclear. The typical approach in children and adults has been a shotgun approach to per-form extensive lab-oratory, radiographic and endoscopic testing in a patient with a cyclic vomiting pattern to exclude an underlying structural, endocrine or metabolic lesion. For example, in a retrospective review of 39 adult patients by Fleischer, multiple studies with normal findings (EGD, UGI and abdominal ultrasound) were obtained on each patient (16). However, based on the relatively low-yield of testing children (27 of 225 = 12%), more cost-effective approaches have been pro-posed. A cost-decision analysis showed that the most cost-effective approach to the initial treatment of children with cyclic vomiting pattern is to make a tentative diagnosis of CVS, perform a single UGI radiograph to exclude malrotation, and begin a two-month empiric trial of anti-migraine medication (26). The upcoming pediatric consensus guidelines (27) on the management of CVS suggest that unless an alarm symptom (Table 5) is present, only a chemistry profile (during the episode) and UGI x-ray to exclude malrotation need be performed initially. However, if alarm symptoms are present or continuous, worsening or nonresponsive symptoms, one should either consider or repeat CT or ultrasound of the abdomen during the episode. There have been no established guidelines for diagnostic evaluation in adults.

TREATMENT

The treatment in CVS is largely empiric and involves a) lifestyle changes, b) prophylactic (antimigraine, anticonvulsant) therapy, c) abortive antimigraine therapy, and d) supportive and symptomatic treatment during episodes. Patients and families are often greatly relieved when the physician identifies CVS as diagnosis and can reassure them that it is not a life-threatening disease. In explaining this mysterious disorder, the physician can draw an analogy to other disabling functional conditions, such as irritable bowel syndrome or even migraines, for which there is no known cause or confirmatory test, but are nevertheless valid diagnoses for which there is reasonable treatment. The physician can then help the family to design a collaborative strategy for preventing and responding to future episodes that will expedite the treatment. Because this disorder is so difficult to treat, a few centers have developed and use a multidisciplinary team featuring a gastroenterologist and nurse, as well as a neurologist and a psychologist.

Recognition and Avoidance of Triggers

A careful history or patient diary can identify triggers such as specific stressors or foods (e.g. chocolate, cheese, MSG) that if avoided may reduce the frequency of episodes. As psychological stress is a well documented trigger in children and adults, psychological counseling and stress reduction techniques may also help. An Australian study reported an association of cyclic vomiting illness with chronic cannabis use with resolution of cyclic vomiting illness after withdrawal from cannabis use (29).

Prophylactic Therapy

Prophylactic therapy taken daily to prevent subsequent episodes has been recommended if the patient has the following characteristics: higher frequency (e.g. >1 episode/month), greater severity (frequent hospitalization), longer duration (e.g. >24 hours) or poor response to abortive therapy. Prophylactic agents include antimigraine medications, anticonvulsants and prokinetics (erythromycin) (30). Antimigraine prophylaxis is more effective in children who have a family history of migraine. In the NASPGHAN Guidelines for children, cyproheptadine is recommended as first line therapy in children <5, and amitriptyline for over five years of age, with propranolol serving as second line (27). These three agents have been shown to decrease the number or severity of episodes by 47%, 75%, and 52% respectively (31). In adults, tricyclic antidepressants (TCA) are the most commonly used agents with amitriptyline doses of up to 100 mg daily required for the desired therapeutic effect. Recently Clouse, et al reported the effective use of levetiracetam or zonisamide as prophylactic agents in adults (32). Other antiepileptics (topiramate) and mitochondrial supplement such as L-Carnitine (33) and Co-enzyme Q10 have demonstrated efficacy in reducing the frequency of migraines and may have a future role in CVS prophylaxis.

Abortive Therapy

Antimigraine medications are used to attempt to terminate breakthrough episodes. Antimigraine triptans, sumatriptan and zolmitriptan both of which can be administered intranasally to circumvent vomiting and loss of oral medication. Sumatriptan, a serotonin (5-HT1B/1D) agonist when administered either by intranasal or subcutaneous route has a 46% efficacy in children (34). Sumatriptan is usually either highly effective and stops the episode completely within two hours or does not alter the episode at all. If that fails, one can proceed to supportive therapy.

Supportive Therapy

Once an acute episode begins or breaks through prophylactic therapy, it usually is refractory to treatment and proceeds along its usual course and duration. The goal is then to reduce the extreme discomfort by attenuating the nausea, vomiting and pain. This management includes reducing stimulation in a quiet, dark room with minimal vital signs because these patients are hypersensitive to light, sound, and even touch. Administration of 5%–10% IV dextrose with NaCl and KCl will correct fluid and electrolyte deficits, hypoglycemia and ketosis 5HT3 antagonist antiemetics such as ondansetron administered at high dose (0.3–0.4 mg/kg/dose ≤25 mg/dose) appear to be much more effective than D2 antagonists (e.g. prochlorperazine) (Table 6). By achieving sleep, sedatives such as lorazepam can further alleviate the unrelenting nausea. For severe pain, either Ketorolac or narcotics (e.g. hydromorphone or morphine) have been used. Often because of the unremitting episodes, these agents are used in combination.

SUMMARY

CVS is an increasingly recognized disorder both in children and adults. Increased awareness of the condition and a high index of suspicion may help decrease delay in diagnosis after symptom onset. A guide is pro-vided here for clinicians who are challenged with the prospect of detecting and evaluating the patient with CVS. Care needs to be delivered by a physician who is somewhat familiar with this disorder and in a nonjudgmental manner. The Cyclic Vomiting Syndrome Association (www.cvsa.online) also provides support with a website, literature, electronic bulletins, phone and email to help children, adults and their families with this difficult disorder. The scarcity of research found in this area indicates further research is needed.

References

1. Li BU, Balint JP. Cyclic vomiting syndrome: evolution in our under- standing of a brain-gut disorder. *Adv Pediatr,* 2000;47: 117-160.
2. Gee S. On fitful or recurrent vomiting. *St. Bart Hosp Rep,*
3. 1882;18:1.
4. Smith PS. Cyclic vomiting and Migraine in children. *Vir Med Month,* 1934;1:591-593.
5. Abu-Arafeh I, Russell G. Cyclical vomiting syndrome in children: a population-based study. *J Pediatric Gastroenterol Nutr,* 1995;21(4): 454-458.
6. Namin F, et al. Clinical, psychiatric and manometric profile of cyclic vomiting syndrome in adults and response to tricyclic therapy. *Neurogastroenterol Motil,* 2007;19(3):196- 202.
7. Li BU, Misiewicz L. Cyclic vomiting syndrome: a brain-gut disorder. *Gastroenterol Clin North Am,* 2003;32(3):997-1019.
8. Boles RG, Adams K, Li BU. Maternal inheritance in cyclic vomiting syndrome. *Am J Med Genet A,* 2005;133(1):71-77.
9. Boles RG, et al. Cyclic vomiting syndrome and mitochondrial DNA mutations. *Lancet,* 1997; 350(9087):1299-1300.
10. Rashed H, et al. Autonomic function in cyclic vomiting syndrome and classic migraine. *Dig Dis Sci,* 1999; 44(8 Suppl):74S-78S.
11. To J, Issenman RM, Kamath MV. Evaluation of neurocardiac signals in pediatric patients with cyclic vomiting syndrome through power spectral analysis of heart rate variability. *J Pediatr,* 1999;135(3):363-366.
12. Taché Y. Cyclic vomiting syndrome: the corticotropin-releasing-factor hypothesis. *Dig Dis Sci,* 1999; 44(8 Suppl):79S-86S.
13. Pfau BT, et al. Differentiating cyclic from chronic vomiting patterns in children: quantitative criteria and diagnostic implications. *Pediatrics,* 1996;97(3):364-368.

14. Li BU, et al. Heterogeneity of diagnoses presenting as cyclic vomiting. *Pediatrics*, 1998; 102(3 Pt 1):583-587.
15. Li BU, Issenman RM, Sarna SK. Consensus statement—2nd Inter- national Scientific Symposium on CVS. The Faculty of The 2nd International Scientific Symposium on Cyclic Vomiting Syndrome. *Dig Dis Sci*, 1999;44(8 Suppl):9S-11S.
16. Tack J, et al. Functional gastroduodenal disorders. *Gastroenterology*, 2006;130(5):1466- 1479.
17. Fleisher DR, et al. Cyclic Vomiting Syndrome in 41 adults: the ill- ness, the patients, and problems of management. *BMC Med*, 2005;3: 20.
18. Prakash C, Clouse RE. Cyclic vomiting syndrome in adults: clinical features and response to tricyclic antidepressants. *Am J Gastroenterol*, 1999; 94(10): 2855-2860.
19. Prakash C, et al. Similarities in cyclic vomiting syndrome across age groups. *Am J Gastroenterol*, 2001; 96(3):684-688.
20. Sato T, et al. Recurrent attacks of vomiting, hypertension and psychotic depression: a syndrome of periodic catecholamine and prostaglandin discharge. *Acta Endocrinol (Copenh)*, 1988; 117(2):189-197.
21. Sato T, et al. A syndrome of periodic adrenocorticotropin and vasopressin discharge. *J Clin Endocrinol Metab*, 1982; 54(3): 517-522.
22. Withers GD, Silburn SR, Forbes DA. Precipitants and aetiology of cyclic vomiting syndrome. *Acta Paediatr*, 1998;87(3):272-277.
23. Forbes D, et al. Psychological and social characteristics and precipitants of vomiting in children with cyclic vomiting syndrome. *Dig Dis Sci*, 1999; 44(8 Suppl):19S-22S.
24. Li BU, Fleisher DR. Cyclic vomiting syndrome: features to be explained by a pathophysiologic model. *Dig Dis Sci*, 1999;44(8 Suppl):13S-18S.

25. Dignan F, et al. The prognosis of cyclical vomiting syndrome. *Arch Dis Child*, 2001; 84(1):55-57.
26. Li BU. Cyclic vomiting: the pattern and syndrome paradigm. *J Pediatric Gastroenterol Nutr*, 1995; 21 Suppl 1: S6-S10.
27. Olson AD, Li BU. The diagnostic evaluation of children with cyclic vomiting: a cost-effectiveness assessment. *J Pediatr*, 2002;141(5):724-728.
28. Li BUK, F. Lefevre., G. Chelimsky, R. G. Boles, S. P. Nelson, D.
29. W. Lewis, S. L. Linder, R. M. Issenman, C. D. Rudolph, The North American Society for Pediatric Gastroenterology, Hepatology and Nutrition. Guideline for the Diagnosis and Management of Cyclic Vomiting Syndrome. 2007; *J Ped Gastroenterol Nutrit*: in press.
30. Tsai JD, et al. Intermittent hydronephrosis secondary to ureteropelvic junction obstruction: clinical and imaging features. *Pedi- atrics*, 2006;117(1):139-146.
31. Allen JH, et al. Cannabinoid hyperemesis: cyclical hyperemesis in association with chronic cannabis abuse. *Gut*, 2004;53(11): 1566-1570.
32. Forbes D. Differential diagnosis of cyclic vomiting syndrome. *J Pediatric Gastroenterol Nutr*, 1995;21 Suppl 1:S11-S14.
33. Li BU, et al. Is cyclic vomiting syndrome related to migraine? *J Pediatric*, 1999;134(5): 567-572.
34. Clouse RE, et al. Zonisamide or levetiracetam for adults with cyclic vomiting syndrome: a case series. *Clin Gastroenterol Hepatol*, 2007;5(1):44-48.
35. Van Calcar SC, Harding CO, Wolff JA. L-carnitine administration reduces number of episodes in cyclic vomiting syndrome. *Clinic Pediatr (Phila)*, 2002;41(3):171-174.
36. Benson JM, Zorn SL, Book LS. Sumatriptan in the treatment of cyclic vomiting. *Ann Pharmacother*, 1995;29(10):9